DERMATOLOGICAL
NURSING AND
THERAPY

DERMATOLOGICAL NURSING AND THERAPY

R.H.SEVILLE MD FRCP
Consultant Dermatologist
Beaumont Hospital
Lancaster

E.MARTIN
Senior State Enrolled Nurse
Beaumont Hospital
Lancaster

Blackwell Scientific Publications

OXFORD   LONDON   EDINBURGH
BOSTON   MELBOURNE

© 1981 by
Blackwell Scientific Publications
Editorial offices:
Osney Mead, Oxford OX2 0EL
8 John Street, London WC1N 2ES
9 Forrest Road, Edinburgh EH1 2QH
52 Beacon Street, Boston
  Massachusetts 02108, USA
214 Berkeley Street, Carlton
  Victoria 3053, Australia

First published 1981

Printed and bound in
Great Britain by
Butler & Tanner Ltd
Frome and London

DISTRIBUTORS

USA
  Blackwell Mosby Book Distributors
  11830 Westline Industrial Drive
  St Louis, Missouri 63141

Canada
  Blackwell Mosby Book Distributors
  120 Melford Drive, Scarborough
  Ontario M1B 2X4

Australia
  Blackwell Scientific Book Distributors
  214 Berkeley Street, Carlton
  Victoria 3053

British Library
Cataloguing in Publication Data

Seville, R. H.
  Dermatological nursing and therapy.
  1. Dermatologic nursing
  I. Title   II. Martin, E.
  610.73'6   RL125

ISBN 0–632–00549–1

Contents

Preface, vii

1. Dermatological nursing, 1

2. Psychosomatic dermatology, 7

3. Psoriasis, introduction to dressings, 12

4. Eczema, infantile eczema, 39

5. Prurigo, neurotic excoriations, artefacts, trichotillomania, alopecia areata, lichen planus, 48

6. Seborrhoeic dermatitis, acne, rosacea, anogenital pruritus, 57

7. Urticaria and drug eruptions, 69

8. Dermatitis, 76

9. Immunology, blistering diseases, 91

10. Cutaneous manifestations of systemic disease and malignancy, 100

11. Granulomata including syphilis, 106

12. Infections—bacterial, fungal and viral, 112

13. Infestations, 135

14. Leg ulcers, 143

v

15. Some problems in the elderly, 156

16. Tumours—benign and malignant, 162

17. Procedures—biopsy, therapeutic and cosmetic, 178

18. Investigations—histological, mycological and bacteriological, 189

19. PUVA, X- and Grenz-ray therapy, physiotherapy, chiropody, dietetics, 192

20. The dermatology team, 200

21. Structure, function and care of the skin, nails and hair, 205

22. Principles of physical treatment and preparations to avoid, 209

Appendix. Dermatological formulary, 215

Index, 221

Preface

This book is for those interested in dermatological nursing and therapy. It aims to be readable rather than exhaustive and presents a practical approach to therapy. The content has been based upon postgraduate courses for nurses and doctors over many years; it forms the basis for the current Joint Board of Clinical Nursing Studies course and is recommended by them as an outline for future dermatology courses. In a short book illnesses have to be classified into artificially watertight compartments which do not occur in nature and dogmatic statements may be made because space is limited. Reference books, such as Rook, Wilkinson and Ebling's *Textbook of Dermatology*, should be consulted for greater detail about the physical and diagnostic aspects of an individual or rare problem.

The fascination of dermatology is that the nurse and physician have an opportunity to observe an illness in its entirety; its physiology, psychology and pathology can be studied more readily than in other disorders, and the correct therapy arranged. Medical science is developing fast and patients tend to be regarded merely as cases; it is the nurse–patient and doctor–patient relationships that suffer most. As will be shown, these relationships are not only complementary to scientific dermatology; they are totally inseparable. The book also aims to demonstrate the simplicity and essence of the various dermatological manifestations in illness and of the nursing therapy that should be given.

Most general nursing books emphasise the connection between mind and body; this is probably because nurses have a close relationship with the patient and inevitably make their own observations. Certain scientific dermatologists argue that it is sometimes difficult to prove stress as a precipitating cause of an illness, and that it is therefore safer not to rely on stress as a factor in case some physical cause is overlooked. Our experience has taught us that both points of view are correct; treatment is only effective when all the aspects of the illness receive attention.

Some illnesses are psychosomatic and some are physical, but often both causes are operative at the same time. This book has been written as a spectrum from the psychosomatic to the physical. Common conditions have been introduced earlier than the rarities; the last mentioned have been included to illustrate certain aspects of pathology and when nursing management is all important. Nursing and therapy have been concentrated upon.

Many of the systemic and other illnesses described have an immunological basis, so a summary of this fast-developing subject has been included at the beginning of Chapter 9. As the structure and function of the skin are dealt with in general training, these subjects have only been covered towards the end of the book, for reference as required.

The 'pen-pictures' of patients have been abridged from their case histories; two are from student days. They have been set as inserts for ease of recognition and are included for emphasis and to stimulate interest.

Acknowledgements

We would like to thank the many who have helped us, and in particular Dr M. H. Seville, Dr G. B. Walker, Mr J. D. Bellis, Mrs H. M. Seville, Miss P. Young and the Dermatological Nursing Team at Beaumont Hospital, Lancaster.

We are grateful to Dr F. T. Madge and the editor of the *Lancet* for permission to reproduce on page 156 the descriptive case history from the 'Peripatetic Column' in 1973 on page 1019, and to the editor of the *Practitioner* for Fig. 2 published in 1977 on page 834.

The late Professor J. T. Ingram's teachings have greatly influenced the patient management described in the book.

We are fortunate to have been able to select photographs from Rook, Wilkinson and Ebling (1979) *Textbook of Dermatology*, 3rd edition, and Solomons (1977) *Lecture Notes on Dermatology*, 4th edition. We are sincerely grateful to the editors, to their contributors and to the publishers Blackwell Scientific Publications.

The following figures have been taken from Rook *et al*: Figs. 13 (38.6), 16 (13.2), 17 (12.17), 18 (12.25), 24 (55.30), 26 (7.6), 28 (54.13), 29 (29.1), 31 (14.10), 32 (14.24), 33 (14.25), 34 (14.13), 37 (14.30), 38 (42.16), 41 (28.1), 43 (61.23), 45 (65.1), 50a–d (24.12), 51 (20.9), 52a & b (20.23), 54 (20.5a), 55 (61.5), 56 (27.16), 57 (33.6), 58 (32.4), 63 (58.12), 64 (66.28), 65a & b (66.47a & e), 66 (66.44), 67 (47.8), 68 (47.10), 70a & b (70.1).

The following figures are taken from Solomons: Figs. 25 (19), 30 (25),

35 (5), 36 (5), 39 (42), 40 (41), 48 (27), 49 (54), 60 (70), 61 (57), 74 (1).

The following colour plates are taken from Solomons: Plates 13 (7), 14 (10), 20 (28), 21 (13), 24 (24), 25 (25), 26 (23), 27 (22), 31 (34).

The numbers in parentheses indicate the Figure number in the original publication. The remaining photographs are either our own or from the Department of Medical Illustration at the Royal Lancaster Infirmary.

R. H. Seville   *Lancaster 1980*
E. Martin

Chapter 1. Dermatological nursing

Nursing is a mixture of compassion and caring for patients, together with scientific knowledge of the illness from which they suffer and its effective treatment. The ability to nurse well comes from experience, patience, kindness—and really caring. It is, a matter of giving oneself to a situation, rather than thinking about what one can get out of it. In caring for patients, confidence develops if there is knowledge and experience of the speciality involved; caring and confidence are a nurse's greatest attributes.

To be effective, nurses and doctors must work as a team, each having knowledge of the other's activities and spheres of influence. Each reinforces the other's work. Much quicker results follow when the doctor prescribes and the nurse treats with confidence. Both must believe in and thoroughly understand the treatment and its method, and convince the patient accordingly. The patient will then have confidence that the team will succeed in clearing his condition. This faith in the team is all-important.

Nurses must always be proficient with dressing and bandaging techniques, and those appropriate to dermatological conditions are detailed on page 32, using psoriasis as an example. Efficiency and attention to detail inspire confidence. The patient can best learn the treatment from example and later be able to look after himself.

In dermatology, nurses are possibly the most important persons in the medical team. They are so much closer to the patient, whether on the ward, or in the home or factory. Patients come to understand and trust them and so they become the main line of communication and feedback for the team, spending much of their time in giving reassurance and carrying out therapy. Time spent talking is never wasted as it provides opportunity for observing the patient as a whole individual.

Rashes that can be precipitated by *psychological* factors are described in the first part of the book. Those caused by *physical* factors, which may be external or internal, are given in the second part.

Nursing management must be based on an accurate medical

1

diagnosis. This can only come from the study of the psychological and social background of an illness, together with the recognition of any physical factors. The diagnosis is finally made from a balanced summing-up of what has been discovered from a full history and examination:

> He looked upset when he mentioned his late wife. A rash had broken out each time within a week after the anniversary of her death, on three separate occasions. It had started on the backs of the hands, particularly the right one, and spread to the skin round the eyes. By now he was crying.

Since examination of the skin must include the normal as well as the affected areas, this was undertaken by the doctor while the nurse comforted him. The history superficially suggested a grief reaction, but the rash looked as if it was produced by external factors to which he was allergic. It transpired that each year he had faithfully placed some chrysanthemums on her grave; his voice nearly broke when he said that they were her favourite flower. The diagnosis of contact dermatitis was confirmed by positive patch test to chrysanthemum leaf. No further attacks occurred after he was told to ask a friend to handle the flowers in future. The advantage in dermatology is that the skin is accessible for all to see; one can observe the effect of any setback, or the obvious improvement when therapy is effective.

The allocation of one nurse to one particular patient is rewarding for both, and a good relationship can then be established. It helps to overcome the patient's natural embarrassment at having to undress for full examination or treatment. The nurse should be relaxed and cheerful, and a gentle sense of humour is invaluable. Patients should be encouraged to understand their treatment and therefore gain confidence in their own ability to look after themselves. Relatives should also be encouraged to understand the treatment and to apply ointment to areas that the patient cannot reach. Seeing and feeling the rash gives greater understanding to both partners with less chance of it forming a barrier between them.

Patients are individuals, with problems and fears, physical defects, and distinctive personalities. The major component of their illness can be classified and treated accordingly, though it must not be assumed that a diagnostic label automatically implies the use of a certain remedy. There must be therapy for the whole patient and his situation, not just the physical treatment of an illness. The term *therapy* covers the physical and the psychological, faith and suggestion, and the use of specific *treatments*. The nurse and doctor must recognise and deal with the many contributing factors for the effects of therapy to be lasting. Patients should be accepted as the fallible human beings they are; if they did not have problems, they would not be patients. They never fail to surprise you; they always do the unexpected! Their needs, reactions and fears must be understood. Those who do not cooperate should not be scolded, but patiently questioned as to what is going wrong, and why. Those with unresolved upsets, instead of accepting them, may project their failure on to the nurse, doctor, or treatment; alternatively they may overtreat themselves, do nothing, or request alternatives.

Most challenges of life evoke a response in the form of appropriate action. This is part of natural development. It is when the challenge becomes too great for the individual to cope with that stress arises and illness may follow. Sometimes the stress is a major event or sometimes it is the summation of many, some of which may seem trivial to the outsider. Stress in a patient requires an outlet. When the outlet is expressed physically the area affected is called the 'target organ'. Due to genetic factors, the part of the anatomy involved varies between families, as for example in peptic ulceration, anxiety states, or in skin affections such as eczema or psoriasis. A genetic tendency cannot be altered, but much can be done to help patients avoid the circumstances that precipitate or worsen an eruption, as will be described later. Treatment of the symptoms alone, as opposed to comprehensive therapy and management, may simply produce a change in target organ:

> She was first seen by one of the team when she was 19; her vulval
> psoriasis had improved with symptomatic treatment, but then an anxiety
> state had developed. The two illnesses had alternated over the years,
> being temporarily helped first by one specialist and then by the other.
> It was when she was 42 that she returned for help. When asked, 'What
> was it that upset you when you were 19?' there was an enraged cry of,
> 'I was jilted', followed by floods of tears. Therapy was then truly effective
> for the first time for 23 years.

Therapy depends on the patient effectively removing or coming to terms with the underlying causes of the condition, together with full dermatological treatment. It includes assessing how the patients are reacting to their environment, and the significance of events in their personal history. Family and personal relationships, home and work are important areas to an adult. Children may react with jealousy to the arrival of another baby, as they are no longer the centre of attention, or have problems at school due to bullying or homesickness. Competitive examinations cause stress at any age.

Therapy should be given as soon as the diagnosis is established, as the prognosis is significantly better when the trouble is dealt with at an early stage. It is important that therapy is continued until the skin is completely clear, as this greatly reduces the chance of any relapse; the result is much less satisfactory when treatment has only been used on an occasional basis to control symptoms, and especially after the rash has been neglected for a period of time.

Chronicity can only be prevented if all aspects of therapy are checked each time the patient is seen. Does the patient understand and accept the psychological and avoid the physical factors causing the rash? Are the local treatments being used correctly and in sufficient quantities, with supplies in reserve? Frequent consultations are sometimes required to achieve the desired effect.

Nervously inflamed skins are worsened by strong antiseptics, which are only required for surgical procedures. Mild cleansers can be used gently, however, so that improvement can be assessed; cleansing too frequently is as counter-productive as inspecting the roots of a plant to see if they are growing!

Tranquillisers are helpful in reducing stress, particularly on a short-term basis while patients are learning to live with their problems. The drugs are best given in small doses after food in the daytime, with twice the dose at night to ensure sleep and to minimise anxiety and apprehension. Benzodiazepine drugs are commonly used. The antihistamines are helpful on account of their sedative side-effects but there is considerable variation between patients as to the dose required. The antihistamines also have a specific effect on urticaria.

Stress is a major cause of irritation that comes on in 'bursts'. Tranquillisers help to break the vicious circle of itching, scratching or rubbing, and consequent damage to the skin, with subsequent worsening of the irritation. Local preparations that reduce irritation also help to break the vicious circle, but they must not be rubbed too vigorously into the skin, as this action in itself may do more harm than good.

Patients rub with their fingertips or heels, or scratch with their nails. When discovered in the act they should be asked, 'What are you doing?', as the scratching may have become a subconscious habit, and they should be made aware of it. A full explanation should then be given of how scratching worsens irritation and the vicious circle becomes established. Patients may then watch themselves in action, and try to aid their recovery by breaking the circle; conscious control of scratching develops first, and later the patient will do himself less damage unconsciously while sleeping. Topical retreatment should be allowed in order to control bursts of irritation. When patients are unconvinced that they rub and scratch, then the linear marks from heel rubbing, the scratches, the smooth fingertips and the remarkable polish of the nails (Fig. 1) should be pointed out as evidence of their habit.

Local treatments that may be a little strong for a sensitive or inflamed skin should not be applied initially to all the affected areas in case a widespread reaction occurs. Dithranol is a good example of this, and is explained on page 21. The words used in front of the patient are important. One should say that the treatment will be 'started' on a few areas and then extended; on no account should the word 'tried' be used, lest the impression be given that the medical team does not know what they are doing! The patient's confidence in the team should always be encouraged. Carefully explaining just how a rash is going to be cleared may be almost as important as the local treatment itself!

The competence of the team is inversely proportional to the number of medicaments they have to use. If all other aspects of the illness have been attended to, then local treatment can be carried out with a few well-proved and simple remedies. Specific preparations are mentioned under the particular diagnostic headings later in the book. It is better to understand the action of a few treatments than be ignorant of what

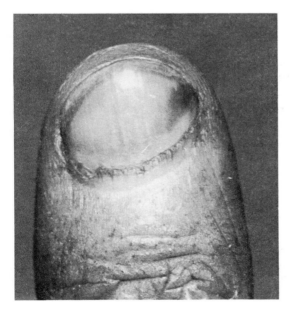

Fig. 1 Fingernail showing polish and bevelling of the edge from frequent scratching.

is happening because the regime is too complicated. Simplicity of method is fundamental and reduces the chance of error. Management of the patient's condition can then be carried out with confidence.

In conclusion it can be said that prescribing remedies is only part of the management of the patient; helping him to understand and avoid the psychological or physical cause of his rash may leave nothing to treat.

Chapter 2. Psychosomatic dermatology

There are those who believe that dermatology should be called 'cutaneous medicine', others favour 'cutaneous psychiatry'! Both are right; all parts of the body are interrelated, the skin reflecting the state of the whole individual. Why is it that in so many specialities an experienced out-patient sister can make a diagnosis more quickly without the numerous investigations that are so often undertaken? She does it by experienced observation of the skin, and seeing whether the patient is medically ill or fundamentally unhappy (Plate 1).

'The eyes are the mirror of the soul: the skin is a canvas on which the psyche reveals itself.'

This statement is not difficult to understand as embryologically the nervous tissue, including the brain, is formed from an infolding of skin a week after conception, when the embryo is only 1.5 mm long. This close relationship between skin and nerves remains throughout life. The simplest example of stress producing a change in the skin is when emotional embarrassment causes nervous vasodilatation of the vessels in the blush area. Kipling wrote, *'the blush that flies at seventeen is fixed at forty-nine.'* Persistent blushing is called rosacea and may be due to stress. The incubation time between the occurrence of stress and its manifestation in the skin is almost instantaneous in the blush, within 2 days in eczema, and within a fortnight in psoriasis:

He was the middle one of three prisoners of war with their heads on execution blocks. His fellows were beheaded. He was sent back to tell the camp to redouble their efforts in building the Thai railway or the same fate would befall them. Extensive psoriasis developed within the week and never cleared. The whole episode was only discovered when he was being treated 30 years later; he woke in the skin ward and had a major abreaction on finding a doctor from the Orient standing at his bedside.

Psychological stress arises when the individual cannot cope with the fact of what has happened. The prisoner of war had suppressed the scene subconsciously for 30 years, causing perpetuation of the rash and chronicity.

Most stress follows problems with interpersonal relationships. When crossing each other's paths in the jungle, animals that are enemies have the options of either flight or fight. The autonomic nervous system prepares for this by metabolising more energy. Civilised behaviour between individuals does not approve of the flight-or-fight response. But when a motorist unexpectedly crosses another's path the autonomic system is just as active!

The effects of stress can be seen in so many different parts of the body; peptic ulceration for example, as well as the skin. It follows that dermatology is much more than 'skin deep'; the speciality cannot be practised by glancing at a rash and just prescribing a remedy. Dermatological disorders account for about 15% of general illness. Despite the large number of patients requiring treatment, it should be emphasised that a conveyor-belt approach will only convince these patients that they are incurable. The full answer to the origin of their problems usually comes from patiently following up the question: 'Apart from genetic reasons, why has this person a rash?'

At consultation, patients will not talk easily about their problems if they are unclothed. On the other hand, before embarking on a long psychological history, it is a great time-saver to make a preliminary examination of the rash to see if it could be due to something obvious, such as scabies! Taking a full and accurate history is important, as in all the other specialities. It must be ascertained that the skin was perfectly clear until a particular time. The area where the rash started, and any spread or variability should be noted. There is a much better chance of obtaining a correct sequence of events if the question of stress is dealt with after all the dates of the history have been carefully recorded. This is because patients may subconsciously suppress the memory of the whole period unless helped to recollect what has happened:

> He was 37 years old, and had developed alopecia areata in February.
> When asked, 'How are your parents?' he answered 'Oh, they are fine.'
> Much time was spent going into interpersonal and work problems but to
> no avail. When again the doctor asked, 'How's your father then?' he
> answered, 'Fine'. 'What about your mother?'—'My God, she died in
> February.'

Consultation is a delicate mixture of experience, intuition, scientific knowledge—and caring. There must be understanding and gentle encouragement, so that the patient feels free to recollect what has happened, the doctor simply acting as a mirror. Recollection of what has happened only comes if there is the right atmosphere—an emotional climate in which the patient feels secure. At no time must there be criticism or impatience.

Recollection can be more readily encouraged when the background is known, as interpersonal problems are the most common cause of stress. If there has been suppression of the memory then the patient should be encouraged to ask his or her partner or parents:

> She was a newly married woman of 20 years of age whose psoriasis developed 4 years previously. She could not recollect anything that upset her just prior to the onset of the eruption and so was told to ask her parents. Both remembered that she had come home almost hysterical one evening after being accosted by a stranger in an unlit country lane. The rash had developed within a fortnight.

It is suppression of the facts and the emotional conflict aroused by an upset that is the main cause of stress, and this suppression may persist as a habit. Habits are normally beneficial as they are a part of learning and therefore time-saving. For example, when learning to drive, the correct sequence and timing with the accelerator and clutch becomes a habit which has to be relearned when changing to automatic transmission. Clinging to the wrong habit may produce amazing and sometimes disastrous results!

When the stress has been recollected by patients, they should be encouraged to accept the upset simply as past history, and not to harbour resentment, self-pity or hurt pride. It is helpful to explain how the memory of an upset can be retained subconsciously in the mind like a habit or, in lay terms, a 'scar on the mind'. This habit perpetuates the stress and therefore the rash. The story of Pavlov's dogs salivating after the ringing of the bell for food is useful to show how the reflex or habit can become established.

Unlike dogs, patients can have the ability to lose their reflex habits if they are willing to see themselves and accept what they may discover. Intelligence and a flexible personality are needed. Firstly they must recall the upset and the associated memories of conflict. Doing so may be a difficult and often emotional experience. At consultation, tears, abreaction or emotional discharge denote release of the repressed stress, which is only possible when there is this insight.

Insight

Insight is defined as self-knowledge: that is, observation and appreciation by the patient of the significance of what has happened, resulting in an understanding in depth and full acceptance; the veneer of superficial recognition only evades real awareness. In other words, there must be complete understanding, acceptance and willingness to relearn and adjust; no longer is the patient being ruled by the effects of old upsets or habits from the past:

> She was 42 years old, but looked younger. Her late husband had been a successful doctor. Maritally she had been very happy. She was worried about finances, the education of the children, and the loss of her partner. A full explanation was given of how stress and worry could be channelled into the skin of her vulval region to produce the irritation and eczematisation (pruritus vulvae). Prescriptions were written up for sedatives and a simple cream for frequent use to control the irritation. At review, a few weeks later, she was clear. Enquiry was made as to the efficacy of the treatment, whereupon she replied, 'I hope you won't be cross, but I never had the prescription dispensed; you explained why I had a rash, and in 3 days it had gone.'

The beneficial effects of insight are shown in Fig. 2.

The difference is statistically significant. Only 20% of patients without insight were clear at 3 years compared with 74% with insight. The patients were psoriatics whose first attacks had been completely cleared with dithranol, as detailed in Chapter 3.

The medical team in the community are the first to be consulted after a stressful situation. They may already know the patient's background and have had to deal with the other people involved, and so can encourage recollection and then insight. Insight can develop more easily when the memory for the event is recent and there has been less chance of the stress being ingrained or imprinted on to the patient's

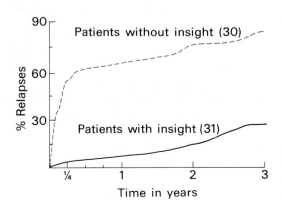

Fig. 2 The prognosis is significantly better in those patients with insight.

mind. Time and patience spent therefore at an early consultation may save a whole lifetime of illness and treatment.

After consultation encouragement and support must be given while the patient is learning to live with what he has just recollected; hence the importance of a close rapport with the medical team. At a later date it is useful to ask, 'Do you understand what pushed out your rash in the first place?' Watch the patient's face while waiting for the reply; blankness, hesitancy or hostility, as well as forgetting or denial, show that there has been no insight. This may be despite having previously recollected the upset at consultation.

The team should be cautious in approaching a longstanding problem, particularly when the patient is inflexible, as is commoner in the older age group. Stress may follow life's challenges, but many of the problems are of the patient's own making, particularly in the interpersonal sphere. In families, one problem leads to another and a vicious circle may be established. Patients and relatives may become so accustomed to an illness that they prefer to blame all their inadequacies on a nasty rash, rather than face up to the problem that caused it. If the rash clears temporarily, then the ointment is given all the credit for the result— or else 'it's the way you put it on, nurse!'.

The nurse will have opportunities of observing the patient in unguarded moments: seeing his joy, irritability, or 'playing to the gallery' when visitors arrive in the ward, or the atmosphere at home when the nurse's visit is not expected. Patients with a subconscious problem often wish to confide in someone they know and trust. There will be an unguarded remark, an innuendo, or the mention of someone out of context who is obviously of great concern to the patient.

Equally important are the gaps in the story where the patient's face becomes blank, as if the shutters have come down; it is then obvious that something has been touched upon that is being hidden from the observer, and probably from the patient himself. Periods of silence will occur if the patient is not yet ready to face up to the problem, and attacks of skin irritation often occur at these moments. Time will then be needed to recall and consider the relevant episodes, whereupon a history interspersed with gaps becomes a logical chain of events.

The continuing repression of an upset is likely to be followed by perpetuation of the rash and chronicity. Who better to prevent this than the doctor and nursing team?

Chapter 3. Psoriasis, introduction to dressings

Psoriasis is one of the most common skin disorders. With rare exceptions it is neither serious nor infective, but can be very embarrassing. It can be so mild that the rash is occasionally observed only as an incidental finding. It may improve during the summer months or in the tropics, but a minority of patients react adversely to sunlight. The condition is less common in the Negro and in warmer climates. Both sexes are equally affected, the disorder becoming apparent any time between 1 and 80 years of age, but mainly in adolescence.

Two to three percent of the British population are affected, but a higher proportion have the genetic predisposition to this condition, as the mode of inheritance is mainly multifactorial. The condition is

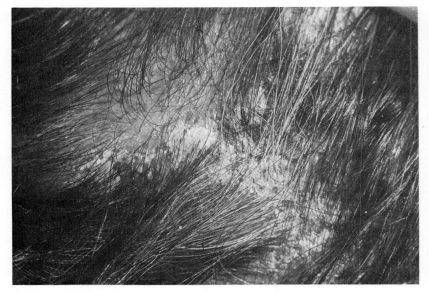

Fig. 3 Psoriasis of scalp showing localised scaly areas.

related to an increase in specific genetic linked antigens (HLA: C17, DMA, B13, BW16, BW17 to date). The predisposition, which of course cannot be altered, is of far less importance than secondary factors which mainly determine the outcome; these can best be alleviated by early therapy as will be described.

Psoriasis is considered to be due to reduced control of epidermal cell division by the central regulating mechanism which are probably in the hypothalamus. The epidermal cells are greatly increased in number and this accounts for the thickness of the lesions which, in the white races, are characteristically salmon pink. The lesions are well-defined papules and plaques and are surmounted by a heap of scales. Air spaces in the basket-weave layer reflect the light causing the characteristic silver appearance of the scales. These tend to be smaller than the lesion which has a smooth, red, well-demarcated edge (Plate 6). Pin-point haemorrhages can be seen if an area is scraped. Psoriatic scales, anchored by hair, become thickly heaped into distinct, firm lesions on the scalp (Fig. 3), which tend not to crumble when touched.

Psoriasis arising at the site of an injury is called the 'Koebner phenomenon' and occurs during a period of extending psoriasis or when new areas are appearing. It is therefore logical that the typical distribution is on the extensor aspects of the knees and elbows (Fig. 4), although it can occur anywhere on the body. The scalp is often involved and in obese women the folds of the axillae, groins and under the breasts, particularly in seborrhoeic subjects.

There are five main presentations:

1 Guttate psoriasis (drop-like) occurs particularly in the younger age group, and often after stress or a streptococcal throat infection; a shower of small lesions occurs all over the body. The scaling is minimal for the first few days. The prognosis is usually good, and only weak treatments are needed. The lesions may progressively enlarge to form the next presentation.

2 Nummular psoriasis (coin-like) is the commonest form and is composed of discs and plaques (Plate 6), especially on the extensor aspects of the limbs and on the trunk.

3 Flexural psoriasis involves the groins (Plate 3), axillae, submammary and other body folds.

4 Localised pustular psoriasis is composed of firm, sterile opaque pustules and their dried brown remnants (Fig. 5). They are present on the palms and soles, with or without the presence of the usual rash elsewhere; fairly strong treatments are usually needed.

5 Approximately one-third of all psoriatics have typical pin-point pits of some or all of the nails (Fig. 6). Larger pits are less common, as

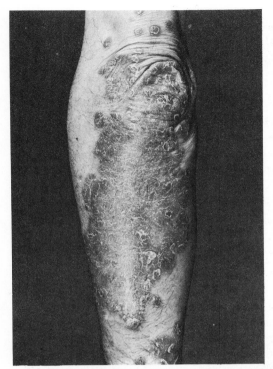

Fig. 4 Psoriasis showing localised plaques.

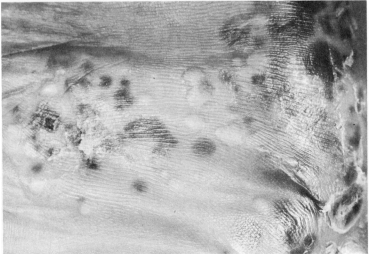

Fig. 5 Pustular psoriasis of sole showing sterile opaque pustules and their dried dark remnants.

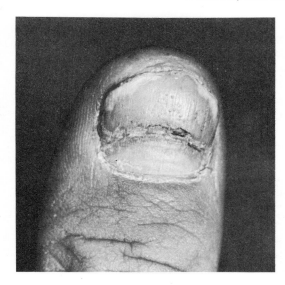

Fig. 6 Psoriasis of nail showing pin-point pits, and a transverse line related to a violent family quarrel two and a half months previously.

is separation of the nail from its bed; this is called 'onycholysis', is usually brown in colour and starts from the centre of the nail plate.

Psoriatic arthritis

Psoriatic arthritis is seronegative and involves the fingers, particularly the terminal joints, and the spine and sacroiliac joints. The nails are often affected first and this makes the diagnosis easier. The skin near the affected terminal joints may also be involved. Usually the skin and joints relapse and remit together, and in these instances therapy for the patient and his skin often helps the joints.

Generalised exfoliative psoriasis

Generalised exfoliative psoriasis is a rare variant which involves the entire skin of the body. The scaling is very much finer but in Caucasians the salmon colour is usually still evident. Sheets of pustules are sometimes present and then it is called generalised pustular psoriasis. It is often a side-effect from the use of strong steroids. Management is described later but emergency admission to hospital should be arranged to prevent hypothermia and loss of body fluid and protein.

Differential diagnosis

The differential diagnosis usually concerns conditions which may overlap or coexist with psoriasis. When occurring on the scalp, face (Plate 1) or flexures, it has more substance and remains more localised than seborrhoeic dermatitis, described on page 57; in the flexures it retains its characteristic colour but the surface is usually smooth and the scaling quite fine. The distribution of the lesions is different from that of eczema, described on page 40, but chronic lichenified patches can be similar in both conditions. Lichen planus has to be suspected if the colour is more violaceous, if any shiny polygonal papules are seen, or if the mouth is affected, as mentioned on page 55. Psoriasis between the toes and of the nails may look like a fungus infection, and so scrapings and clippings may have to be sent for microscopy and culture before making the diagnosis.

Secondary factors

Secondary factors can precipitate or exacerbate psoriasis. Physical ones include tonsillitis or intercurrent infections (10% of sufferers) and may also occur with changes in hormone levels, as during puberty and the menopause. It is rare for psoriasis to develop during pregnancy; usually it improves and can even clear, often worsening after confinement. Mitigating any of these secondary factors improves the prognosis: for example, penicillin VK is helpful when the patient has a persisting streptococcal infection. However, a low dosage is given (as in the prevention of rheumatic fever), its effect being monitored by throat swabs and the antistreptolysin titre.

  Psychological stress is an important secondary factor. In a research series at least half the first attacks were found to have been precipitated by an episode of considerable emotional involvement. Many were of an interpersonal nature and from within a family group. There was significantly less stress of a similar degree in a control series. The interval between an episode of stress and the first appearance of the rash (incubation time) was within a fortnight in two-thirds of the instances:

A wife's intractable psoriasis, predominantly of the face and vulval region, appeared within 10 days of finding her husband in bed with his girlfriend.
One schoolboy had his first attack when taking the 11 plus exam and had recurrences at 'O' level, 'A' level, and university finals. His parents were ambitious for him.
A man's extensive psoriasis developed within 2 days of being torpedoed and sunk twice in one wartime convoy.

Prognosis

The prognosis is improved when the time between the onset and clearance is short, or when a secondary factor is found and treated such as infection or stress. It is improved when there is insight and also when the time taken to clear the eruption is short. Complete clearance of the rash is essential before the prognosis can be favourably altered; this cannot be emphasised too forcibly.

Psychological management

Psychological management involves therapy for any secondary factors; if this is combined with physical treatment, patients can be completely cleared and kept clear for periods measured in years. The family doctor and community nurse are in the privileged position of being the first persons to be consulted. At this stage there will be a greater chance of helping the patient recollect an upsetting incident, especially if it is of recent origin:

> She was an attractive lady of 20, with full-length auburn hair, fair complexion and quite a high octane rating! Extensive psoriasis had developed within a fortnight of discovering that her lover was married. It involved her face, anogenital region and round the breasts. The doctor helped her gain insight into how the rash had been caused. Relief from irritation was within days and improvement in the rash took place within a fortnight. Local treatment with a weak dithranol preparation was all that was needed to completely clear the eruption.

Teaching the patient to understand and accept his problems is as important as making sure he learns the physical treatment. Once taught how to look after themselves correctly, patients will gain confidence that the therapy will be equally effective if needed in the future. Any minor flare-ups which occur will then assume far less importance and can be quickly dealt with, often without seeing a doctor.

When the eruption is either extensive or longstanding, treatment is best carried out initially in special centres by fully trained staff and where the reputation for success stimulates the faith of the patient. This also provides a good opportunity for contact between nurse and patient, during which important observations and assessment can be made. Much vital information can be gathered to back up or adjust the doctor's assessment of the psychological factors in the patient's condition. This is easier on the ward, which has the added advantage that the patient is temporarily shielded from his problems. Admitting patients at the beginning of the week enables any difficulties or reactions to treatment to be sorted out before the weekend when consultant supervision is not so readily available.

Patient allocation

Patient allocation, where a particular nurse is assigned to carry out most of the treatment for a particular patient, is a development which has proved very beneficial in the treatment of psoriasis, as well as in other skin conditions. It strengthens the nurse–patient relationship and helps to reduce any of the patient's embarrassment. This continuity also means that the nurse quickly learns to control the treatment. Of great importance is pride in her work. Enthusiasm is infectious. Both nurse and patient obtain great satisfaction in seeing the rash disappear. A sense of humour is essential to overcome the patient's embarrassment from the presence of the psoriasis and also from being handled during its treatment. When opportunity presents, laugh with the patient. If a particular area causes embarrassment, delicately joking about it often helps.

A patient often requires encouragement to get better. The nasty rash, that alienates him from the family, can be used as an excuse for not facing up to relationships that may have gone wrong, or the fact of their absence. Even in failure everyone has their pride:

> He was 55 years of age and had married late. His wife, who was 35, had left him to live with a younger man to whom she was madly attracted. It was amazing how well the husband had coped with the children, as well as holding down his job at the same time. The wife found that a true relationship cannot be based solely on sex, even though this was the first time she had ever enjoyed it. She returned to look after the children, but demanded a bedroom to herself. It was then that he developed psoriasis. Treatment was only effective when the wife was ultimately persuaded to care for him by touching and undertaking the treatment of the back and scalp, where he could not reach or see so effectively.

Relatives should be taught how to treat the rash and helped to understand how it originated. Their physical contact during treatment gives support and confidence to the patient, as does meeting other patients with similar problems and rashes; seeing these cleared shows that it can be done!

Because lay people unfortunately find rashes loathsome, patients can at least guarantee to get a seat to themselves on the bus! They find that physical contact is reduced or avoided even by close relatives. Make a point therefore of shaking hands and touching patients while carrying out treatment. It is very important that the nurse handles the skin confidently and without reluctance or the artificial barrier of gloves. This absence of gloves also enables her to make a much more accurate assessment of the skin's return to normality; just as important, treatment can be localised very accurately and the amounts applied carefully controlled. Fingerstalls provide a compromise (Fig. 7a) to avoid staining the nurses fingernails. Otherwise gloves are only needed when there is secondary infection with pathogenic organisms, as described later in the chapter on leg ulcers, though not all dermatologists feel that this is necessary.

Tranquillisers are useful during the period when the patient is facing up to what has actually happened; they are helpful when there is pruritus which is usually a sign of tension. They also reduce the incidence of fresh patches or 'sprouts' of psoriasis during treatment, due to the continuing unresolved upset. These may occur following a visit by relatives or friends, or simply following the doctor's attempt to help the patient develop insight. Nurses have good opportunity to watch for this.

Patients with unresolved psychological problems may overtreat themselves, or on the other hand blithely claim how diligent they are, when the skin shows untreated silvery scales with no dithranol stain whatsover! Sometimes they become intolerant to the antipsoriatic remedies; alternatively, they may resist the physical action of the treatment in the same way that a devout Fakir can walk on hot coals!

Although undue preoccupation with the eruption often denotes lack of insight, the very presence of the rash may cause real despondency and a feeling of inevitability that nothing can be done, which further worsens the eruption. An accurate history should show whether the despondency has followed rather than precipitated or worsened the psoriasis; it is best dispelled by a confident explanation of what treatment is going to be given, followed by prompt and complete clearance of the eruption.

It is essential to the success of treatment that the nurse has a genuine interest in skin disorders. If the nurse is confident in her ability to treat, the patient in turn will realise that not only is the rash going to get better, but also he will be able to cope with any recurrence of it in the future.

Physical treatment

Once established, psoriasis is a condition that usually requires physical treatment for clearance to take place, and this is why therapy is so worthwhile. Understanding the condition and its treatment gives meaning to routine procedures; it is very easy to forget that a matter of routine to the nurse may require a full explanation to the patient.

The skin must always be treated gently and never rubbed or cleaned roughly, as this will cause further damage. Slack dressings, which have to be constantly readjusted by the patient may also do harm, as well as spreading ointment, causing discomfort and being psychologically detrimental. Dressings should be cut and applied carefully, as described later (see page 32).

A patient with a rash all over the body should not be left completely naked for any longer than necessary while treatment is being carried out. After the rash has been checked, the trunk should be the first area to be treated and then covered with dressing. Next the arms should be treated, then the legs. The anogenital region should be left until last; he is usually sitting on it anyway!

Buttocks may need retreatment if the ointment is wiped off when not lying or sitting still. Cracks in the anogenital region may benefit from retreatment, especially when there is soreness.

The patient and nurse must know how and when to treat, and when to stop. All patients should be given and helped to fully understand a proforma, such as the one appended at the end of this chapter. The secret with local treatment is to obtain the patient's trust and confidence, so that he will diligently follow your instructions.

Psoriasis is due to rapid cell division; the treatment is therefore designed to reduce this and to enable the formation of normal skin. There are two safe and equally effective local treatments: coal tar and dithranol (anthralin). Both have been used with safety for three-quarters of a century. It is unfortunate that attempts to make them cleaner to use by modifying them chemically invariably reduce their effectiveness. Patients however will cooperate with the treatment if the benefits are fully explained, especially the fact that longer periods of clearance follow their use.

Tar is less potent than dithranol and therefore takes longer to act but does not need to be applied accurately. Each treatment has advantages over the other, as will be explained. Dithranol is the better preparation for treatment at home and will be described first. Any regime must be simple so that it can easily be taught, understood and carried out by the patients themselves in the event of a relapse.

Dithranol

Dithranol must not be used on acute spreading psoriasis; bland applications such as yellow soft paraffin or emulsifying ointment are then required. Care is also needed for at least a month after the previous use of strong local steroids, until therapeutic rebound has ceased and the skin has had time to recover. Weak applications are needed for psoriasis that is erupting or spreading (Plate 5), whilst thick indolent patches require stronger preparations (Plate 6). On the sensitive areas such as the flexures, or on thin or guttate psoriasis, treatment should be less frequent or a weaker strength used. It is safer to start on only a few areas in order to assess the response to the treatment, as very rarely patients can be intolerant to it. A few days later, after a satisfactory reaction, the preparation can be extended. Thicker areas should be treated first as they will be the most resistant and the last to clear. The stronger the preparation, the greater the need for accurate application to the lesions (Plates 7–10), and for the ointment base to be stiff in order to prevent spread to normal skin; stiffening the base, as well as resting the affected part after treatment, also enhances the effect. Treatment at home is therefore best done just before bedtime. Advising rest or a period off work is sometimes necessary so that patients can concentrate on clearing themselves. Ward patients should take their physical activity just before treatment rather than just afterwards!

It takes 2–3 days for the full effect of an application to show. It is therefore very much easier for one nurse to judge how much dithranol her individual patient's skin will tolerate, and later to monitor the effects of the treatment, than for several to be involved—a further demonstration of the importance of nurse–patient allocation. Spread of the preparation on to the surrounding skin can be due to slack dressings, the ointment base being too soft, the nurse not applying it accurately, the patient scratching or rubbing it, or not resting after the application. The stronger preparations will burn normal skin and may result in quite unnecessary abandonment of the treatment. Fair-skinned patients are a little more sensitive than dark ones, and there is always the possibility that strong steroids have been used more recently than the patient will admit.

A sensation of slight sunburn should be aimed at by adjusting the frequency of application and the amount applied. Treatment should be suspended for a few days or reduced in strength if there is a sensation of burning. Suspension will have to be longer if the lesions become glazed, especially if there is any moistness, or if there is more than a gradual spread of the psoriasis. A bath should then be taken and yellow soft paraffin applied for a few days; crystal violet 0.5% in water is probably the best preparation for a moist treatment burn. The nurse may be allowed on her own initiative to use this dye as it is a safe preparation and its use is apparent.

Starting with the potent stiff dithranol 0.5% preparation from the onset is a considerable time-saver, but patient and staff must have experience of this technique (Plates 7–10). There is also the advantage that patients can learn its use while thick lesions are still present. This ensures that the patient learns the necessary attention to detail that will ultimately result in a better prognosis. The dithranol requires very accurate localisation to prevent burning of the normal surrounding skin (Fig. 7a, b). It should only be used a few times a week for the treatment of thin lesions. Intelligent patients and particularly those who have marital partners prefer to use a stronger preparation a few times a week, rather than a weaker one on a nightly basis. The weaker preparations are much safer when the patient's ability to carry out the detailed treatment is in doubt.

Dithranol stains the psoriatic areas red-brown. The darker the stain, the greater the improvement. Patients will not carry out treatment properly unless this is explained to them. The treatment must be continued until the skin is entirely clear. It is then completely smooth with nothing to feel on palpation. Gently scratching the areas no longer produces any fine silvery scaling. At this stage the dithranol stains usually peel off, exposing skin of normal colour and patterning. It is important to recognise this stage to ensure full clearance. Treatment must then be stopped to prevent burning the new skin. If strong concentrations are being used and there is any doubt about the skin being perfectly clear, it is safer to continue with a weaker preparation until the skin is completely smooth. The stain disappears about 1 week after cessation of treatment.

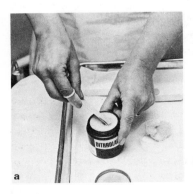 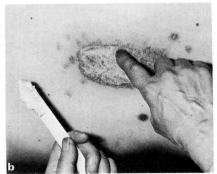

Fig. 7a & b   Accurate application of stiff dithranol ointment to psoriasis of skin. The carrying spatula is thrown away after use.

Ordinary baths are an essential part of any dithranol regime. The skin accumulates the medicament, acting as a reservoir and intensifying its action. A bath should normally be taken before every application in order to control the treatment reaction. Don't let patients scrub the stain off their skin as this delays progress. After the bath, letting the skin dry completely makes it much easier to see which areas still need treating.

Following a satisfactory response, the bath and next application can be postponed, as the dithranol retained in the keratin layer continues to be active. This can considerably reduce the time spent on applying the treatment. In the ward, patients should not bath until the nurse assesses that the psoriasis will tolerate another application of dithranol. By giving patients 1½ hours warning of when to take a bath, the nurse can plan her workload and maximise the ward's resources.

The treatment response can be increased by either reducing the number of baths, or by twice-daily applications of dithranol. Crêpe bandages or microporous rayon adhesive tape (Micropore) can be applied over the ointment on the elbows, knees and thicker areas to aid localisation and increase effectiveness. Plastic adhesive strapping BPC is even more effective but should only be used for short periods as its repeated removal aggravates the surrounding normal skin. Thorough dusting with talcum powder (Fig. 8a, b) and covering with old nylon tights also helps to prevent the ointment spreading. In the tropics, open-leg tights or knee-length stockings are probably the best dressing material for both sexes. Old pyjamas, sheets, pillowcases and underclothing should be used because of the staining. In the ward, disposable or green sheets should be used. Further details of dressings are given later in the chapter (page 32). To avoid staining with dithranol, the nurse should cover her nails and fingers with soft paraffin before giving treatment, and wash off afterwards; any staining can be removed with trichloroethylene or benzene.

Dithranol 0.2% ointment or 0.25% cream are at least four times less potent than the stiff dithranol 0.5% preparations. The weaker dithranol does not require such localisation if only applied on alternate days. It is a useful strength with which to start treatment in order to assess the patient's reactivity, though dithranol 0.1% cream may be used daily instead. The creams are suitable for treatment of the scalp, flexures and sensitive areas. They can be used on the face if localised by microporous adhesive tape (Fig. 9a, b) to prevent the dithranol getting into the eyes and causing conjunctivitis.

The creams are excellent for treatment of the scalp as plenty can be

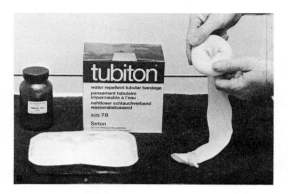

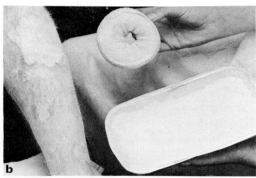

Fig. 8a & b   Making and using a pad to apply talc over stiff dithranol ointment to reduce spreading.

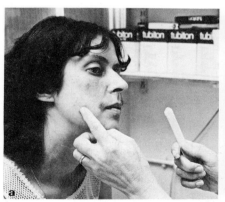

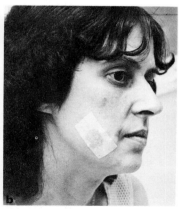

Fig. 9a & b   Psoriasis of face treated with dithranol cream localised by microporous tape.

applied. Dithranol stains silver hair the colour of the rinse called 'Rosewood Accord'; telling female patients this fact may improve the chance of the treatment being carried out! The hair should be shampooed before each application to control the treatment reaction, remove scales and to assess progress. Allow complete drying afterwards, as otherwise it is not possible to identify the areas that are not perfectly smooth and clear. These appear as areas of silvery scales or roughness. Hair dryers should only be used with moderation. Use a comb for inspection and to make it easier to apply the cream directly on to the scalp (Fig. 10). Continue treatment for at least a week after all areas are entirely smooth. Resistant areas may require dithranol 0.5% cream or even the stiff ointment accurately applied. Coal tar and salicylic acid ointment BPC is needed to remove the stiff preparation as it contains no emulsifier. It is important to be able to identify the yellow-brown scales of a drying treatment burn, which should be managed cautiously.

Psoriasis of the external auditory meatus (Fig. 11) is best treated with dithranol 0.25% cream. Initially this should be applied sparingly with a wisp of cottonwool round an applicator; sterile swabs used for bacteriology are too wide and unnecessarily expensive. The treatment response can be regulated by increasing the frequency of application and quantities used as required.

Flexural psoriasis responds to dithranol 0.1% or 0.25% creams usually applied daily. These areas look inflamed and there is the temptation to

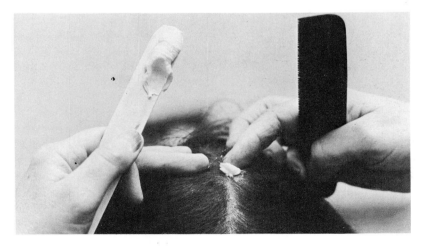

Fig. 10 Psoriasis of scalp being treated with dithranol cream.

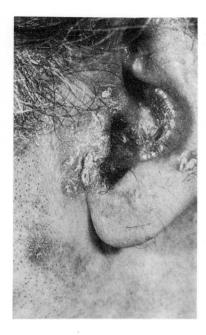

Fig. 11 Psoriasis of
the external auditory
meatus.

reduce or stop the treatment, but then the psoriasis worsens again.
Painful cracks should be treated with crystal violet 0.5% in water.
After this has dried the dithranol should be applied. The soreness may
discourage its use but then neither the crack nor the psoriasis will heal.
Cracks infected with Gram-negative organisms should be treated with
silver nitrate 0.5% in water before the dithranol is applied. Resistant
areas may require the 0.5% cream or even the occasional application
of stiff dithranol 0.5% ointment. Treatment should not be stopped
before the texture of the skin has returned to normal (Fig. 12).

Crude coal tar BPC

Crude coal tar BPC applied daily is a good alternative to dithranol
0.5%; it is better for lichenified psoriasis because of its antipruritic
properties as the thickening of the lesions is mainly caused by constant
rubbing and scratching (Fig. 13). The tar is messy and therefore limited
to hospital use. It gives excellent results when applied after a good
initial dithranol response. Scottish Distiller's Tar is recommended as
being less irritant and therapeutically more effective. It can be easily
removed with one application of coal tar and salicylic acid ointment.

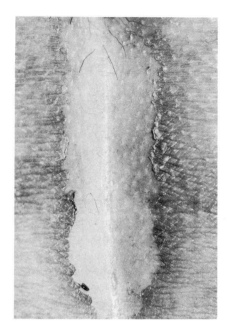

Fig. 12   Flexural psoriasis cleared with dithranol cream, the dithranol stain peeling off to leave normal skin underneath.

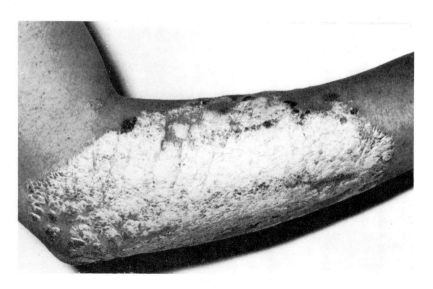

Fig. 13   Lichenified psoriasis following rubbing and scratching.

Tar is best applied with a paintbrush, but these are very difficult to clean. A good alternative is a wooden spatula covered with layers of tubular cotton gauze (Tubiton 01), much as one would apply for a thick protection to a finger (Fig. 14a–d). These are very easy to make and are disposable. Coal tar does not need to be applied accurately, but the finish should be smooth and of equal thickness. Dressings may be applied before the tar dries. Don't use powder, or cracking and peeling will take place. Next day some of the tar is inevitably removed with the dressings, the areas being irregular in shape; linear areas denote continued rubbing or scratching by the patient. The texture of the rash can then be observed in places, and the time when all the tar should be cleaned off for clinical inspection may be estimated. This is best done by softening the tar with an application of coal tar and salicylic acid ointment, followed by a bath the following day. Trauma should be avoided. Out-patients can have the tar covered with adhesive elastic extension plaster. Surrounding hairs should be shaved off beforehand. These dressings last up to a fortnight, provided the patient does not

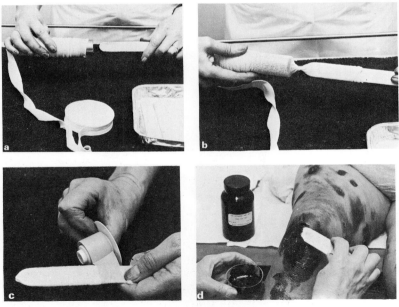

Fig. 14a–d   Making an applicator and applying crude coal tar.

scratch them loose. Resistant psoriasis of the scalp responds well to crude coal tar 30% in emulsifying ointment. Initially this should be applied sparingly and not used if there is any infection. The ointment can easily be removed by shampooing in order to observe the clinical effect.

The main complication of treatment with tar is folliculitis, which is apt to develop in certain individuals after about a week's treatment; its incidence can be reduced by one application of crystal violet 0.5% in water, which should be allowed to dry before the tar is applied. This is important as folliculitis may initiate a Koebner relapse of the psoriasis. Intolerance to tar can occur as a smouldering erythematous reaction which rapidly settles when the strength of the treatment is reduced. Allergic sensitivity to tar is rare.

Stiff dithranol

Stiff dithranol 0.5% ointment is a potent preparation. Salicylic acid is added to prevent deterioration, the ingredients being dispersed in chloroform 2.5% in equal quantities of hard and soft paraffin (candle-wax and petrolatum). It is available as Dithrolan. The dispersal is vital as dithranol is an irritant when not dissolved or milled into the preparation. Accurate localisation of the ointment is needed, as has already been described. It is stiff enough not to spread but convenient to use at home.

Dithranol 0.2% ointment can be prepared most easily by pharmacists diluting 1 part of the 0.5% ointment with 1½ parts of yellow soft paraffin as the dithranol remains well dispersed. Hospital pharmacies can prepare the ointment carefully from the original ingredients.

Zinc and salicylic acid paste BP (Lassar's Paste) provides a suitable alternative base for dithranol, but the preparation is not as convenient to use at home. The paste needs to be specially prepared in order to disperse the dithranol, and is therefore only available from hospital pharmacies. It deteriorates on storage. Nurses accustomed to pastes should use only *half* the amount of the stiff dithranol ointment and apply it *half* as frequently, as the ointment is more potent and quicker in action than the paste. This is even more important when the stronger dithranol concentrations are used. Mention should be made of the importance of simplifying any hospital regime so that once taught, patients can carry out the treatment of relapses at home. Dithranol creams and stiff ointments are much better than pastes for this purpose.

Ointments or pastes are always more effective than creams as they hydrate the skin and have a greater depot effect; the difference is especially noticeable when the psoriatic scales are thick. Ointments are quicker to apply and should be used when nurses are carrying out the treatment; creams are much better for patients to apply—because of their convenience they actually get used! Creams are really effective for the treatment of flexures and scalps, as plenty can be applied and a satisfactory response obtained. Surplus dithranol cream left on the skin causes staining of clothing or dressings. It therefore has to be applied more sparingly and smoothed into the skin until no surplus remains. Old night clothing can then be worn followed by normal clothing the following day. Dithranol creams are available in 0.1%, 0.25% and 0.5% strengths.

Coal tar and salicylic acid ointment BPC is useful in the treatment of psoriasis on the scalp and face, during weaning from topical steroids, and in acute spreading psoriasis. It is rather weak and requires no localisation. Mainly because it is greasy, it is excellent for softening heaped scales in the scalp before they can be removed by shampooing; dithranol creams can then be effective.

Zinc and coal tar paste BPC (White's Tar Paste) is a useful and more effective alternative to coal tar and salicylic acid, but is cosmetically less acceptable, containing three times more tar. It is about as effective as dithranol 0.1% ointment and may irritate areas which have previously reacted to strong treatment. Cooking oil makes removal of the paste easier.

White's Tar Paste is also useful in the very few patients who are truly intolerant to dithranol. It requires no localisation and can therefore be used daily by patients who cannot be relied upon not to overtreat themselves! It is probably the best preparation for removing dithranol stains. This can be undertaken when patients are anxious to have the stain removed, or if there is any doubt that the psoriasis is completely clear; indeed for these reasons, some in-patient units use White's Paste for half a week towards the end of their dithranol regimes.

It is unwise to prescribe less effective antipsoriatic ointments, such as salicylic acid 5% for stain removing, except for short periods only; as they are less messy, patients will use what remains of the preparation for the treatment of relapses instead of the dithranol which is far more rapid and effective. In the same way, steroids must not be used in conjunction with tar or dithranol regimes, as the patients will choose the cleaner but purely suppressive preparation.

Yellow soft paraffin (petroleum jelly, petrolatum) has no active ingredients, but is useful as an alternative to coal tar and salicylic acid ointment in bringing symptomatic relief during weaning from steroids, in acute spreading psoriasis, and temporarily following inadvertent burns by dithranol.

Other treatments

Tar baths and conventional *ultraviolet light* although traditional, have been found to have little long-term effect; they detract from the more important aspects of management, just as in the use of pastes that cannot be easily applied at home. Lack of facilities is then used as an excuse for not carrying out the local treatment in the event of relapse.

Topical steroids would have a place in the treatment of psoriasis if doctors could predict which patients would clear spontaneously. The steroids are clean and easy to use, but unfortunately are only suppressive in action; withdrawal is quickly followed by relapse and even potentially dangerous side-effects. Dependence may occur, along with telangiectasia, atrophy and permanent striae, and absorption resulting in adrenocortical suppression. Generalised exfoliative and pustular psoriasis are very rare in districts where strong topical or systemic steroids are not used for psoriasis; widespread unstable psoriasis (Plate 4) is also much less common.

Weaning a patient who has become dependent on potent steroids is very difficult. As soon as the preparation is stopped, the rash worsens in the form of a therapeutic rebound. The unstable skin will then only tolerate a bland application until it has recovered. Methotrexate or Grenz rays, described on page 195, are helpful during this period.

Methotrexate and other cytotoxic drugs are also useful additions in the treatment of severe cases of psoriasis. They reduce the cellular-proliferation, but have potentially dangerous side-effects which have to be carefully monitored, and this includes a liver biopsy. The kidneys, liver, testes and blood-forming organs are most at risk. Patients should avoid alcohol in case cirrhosis is developing, and conception for half a year after taking the drug as it is potentially teratogenic. The benefits of the treatment must always be weighed against the risks and the drug continued no longer than necessary.

Methotrexate is very effective in severe disabling and in generalised exfoliative psoriasis, in reducing the activity of the rash, and enabling earlier introduction of local antipsoriatic preparations. Grenz rays are equally effective. Initially bland applications such as yellow soft paraffin, emulsifying ointment, or Boots E45 cream are needed. Approximately a week later, very weak dithranol, such as 0.05% to

0.1% in yellow soft paraffin, can then be cautiously introduced on a few thicker areas. The ointment base is more soothing than paste and has the advantage of not needing cleaning off, which is usually a painful procedure. If the response is satisfactory after a week, the treatment can be extended. The nurse and patient are often more enthusiastic about extending the treatment than a cautious doctor! Don't forget that these patients are not fit enough to be bathed. The dithranol should only be increased to 0.2% when this can be carried out. Experience is needed to tell the difference between an exacerbation of the exfoliative psoriasis and treatment intolerance. Exfoliative psoriasis is salmon coloured with fine scales; treatment intolerance is fiery red, glazed or oozing; both are sore and uncomfortable. Previous use of steroids makes the distinction more difficult. Nursing care and encouragement are vital factors in management.

Once the patient is fit enough he should be encouraged to return home for a few days at a time, initially on the weak treatment. Later he can be followed up at out-patients until the psoriasis stabilises itself into patches; strong remedies can then be started.

PUVA is a useful treatment for patients suffering from severe psoriasis, and details are given on page 192. The best results are obtained when it is used as an adjunct to a dithranol regime.

Dressings—an introduction

Dressings are necessary to localise treatment, to prevent applications being rubbed off and for protection of the skin against trauma or scratching. In general the dressings are the same for psoriasis as for other skin conditions. They should be cut accurately and applied carefully. The techniques can only be understood by watching them being done and learned with practice.

There is a full range of tubular cotton gauze, such as Tubiton:

72—adult body. T1—child body, head dressing or large legs.
78—normal legs. 56—arms or thin legs.
34—children's arms. 01—fingers.

Applicators are unnecessary, except for fingers and tend to over-stretch the dressings. If required, further support and protection for areas such as the knees and elbows can be given by a layer of crêpe bandage over the tubular gauze. If this technique is used, knots in the gauze will be unnecessary.

The trunk

The trunk requires T1 or T2, to form a body stocking (Fig. 15a–d). It must be cut long enough to reach down to the mid-thigh, so as to afford protection to any treated area of the buttocks. It should be folded in half in a vertical plane, and an almost vertical incision (Fig. 15c) made through the outer edges for the arms; if the incision is more horizontal there will be a gap in the protective covering, in front of and behind the arms. Making an incision lower down will enable the neck to be protected (Fig. 15d).

The arms

The arms require Tubiton 34 or 56. A single longitudinal cut (Fig. 15e) in the dressing under the axilla enables it to be tied to the one from the other side, in front and behind the neck (Fig. 15g). At the lower end, a single longitudinal cut should be made up to the end of the area to be covered, the dressings turned back, and holes cut for the thumb, middle and little finger as required (Fig. 15h). The spare should be tied round the wrist.

The fingers

The fingers should be dressed with Tubiton 01, when localisation of the treatment is needed (Fig. 15i); cotton gloves tend to spread the applications. Two layers should be applied to each finger, twisting the dressing

Fig. 15a–s Tubular gauze dressings.

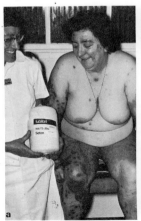 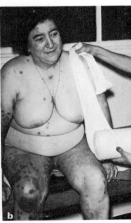 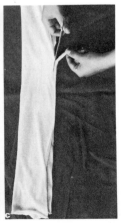

(a) Patient–nurse relationship (E.M.)

(b) Measuring for the trunk

(c) The gauze is folded in half and then cut almost vertically for the arms

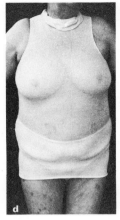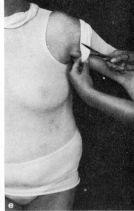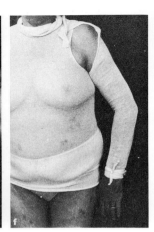

(d) Making the incision
lower down means the
neck is protected

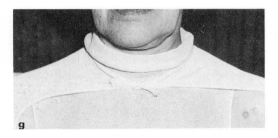

(e–g) A longitudinal
cut in the arm dressing
enables it to be tied to
the one on the other
side

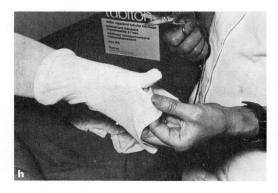

(h) Holes are cut for
fingers as required

on itself at the distal end (Fig. 15j). After a single longitudinal cut (Fig. 15k), the spare gauze can be tied round the wrist (Fig. 15l).

The legs

The legs require Tubiton 56, 78 or T1. It should be long enough to reach from well above the hips to beyond the toes. A single medial longitudinal cut in the gauze should be made at the top of each leg (Fig. 15m), and the spare gauze tied above the hips, in front (Fig. 15n) and behind the abdomen. At the feet, the dressing should be twisted (Fig. 15o), doubled back, another longitudinal incision made over each limb, and the ends of the dressings tied round each ankle (Fig. 15p).

The scalp

It is only necessary to dress scalps when the treatment is really messy. Tubiton T1 can be put on the scalp, twisted at the top and the ends rolled under each other (Fig. 15q).

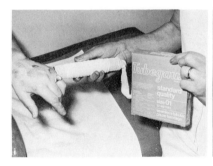
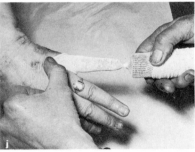

(i–l) Finger dressings

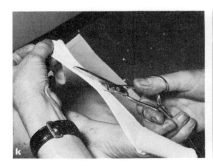
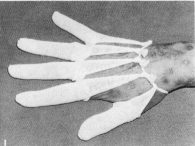

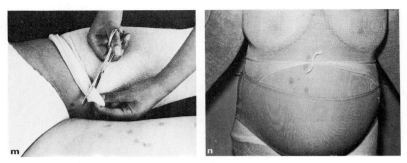

(m–n) The leg dressings are cut and tied round the waist to each other.

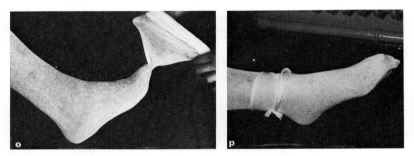

(o–p) The dressing is twisted over the toes, cut and tied off round the ankle.

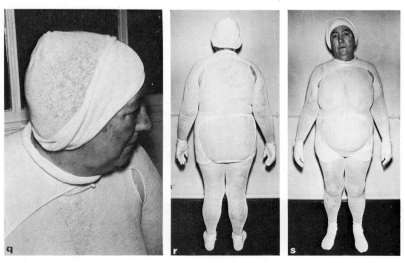

(q–s) Completed dressings.

Psoriasis treatment

Dithranol 0.5% with salicylic acid 0.5% in equal parts of hard and soft paraffin is a potent ointment for accurate use about twice a week on thin psoriasis and daily only on thick psoriasis. (The ointment is commercially available as Dithrolan.) For ease of application in cold weather, keep in a warm place.

1 A bath must be taken before each application because this helps to keep the treatment reaction under control by preventing a build-up of dithranol in the skin.

2 Apply Dithrolan accurately just to the psoriasis (usually before going to bed) starting with a few of the thicker areas first in order to judge the reaction. Aim for a local feeling of warmth. A sensation of burning can be controlled by stopping treatment for a few days, and then resuming with less ointment less often, depending on the patient's individual response. The psoriasis will then become thinner as a red-brown stain develops; *the darker the stain the greater the improvement.* Scrubbing the stain off in the bath delays healing.

A thorough dusting with talc and covering with old nylon tights helps to prevent the ointment spreading on to the surrounding skin. Alternatively applying microporous adhesive tape over the ointment or cream to be described localises and enhances their effect. Because of staining, old pyjamas, sheets and pillowcases, also old underclothing should be used.

3 Alternatively thin lesions and also the flexures can be treated with dithranol 0.25% cream several times a week depending on the response described in 2. It should be smoothed into the lesions until no surplus remains.

4 Scalp: treat affected areas with dithranol 0.25% cream after shampooing usually daily, until the scalp is smooth; then continue less frequently for a further week. The shampoo helps to control the treatment reaction. Resistant areas should be treated with dithranol 0.5% cream, or even the ointment.

5 Face: use dithranol 0.25% cream as per 3 but more sparingly, keeping it away from the eyes. Alternatively use zinc and coal tar paste BPC (White's Paste), which is also useful for removing treatment stains.

The treatment must be continued until the skin is entirely clear. It is then completely smooth with nothing to feel on palpation. Gently scratching the areas no longer produces any fine silvery scaling. At this stage the dithranol stain can be seen peeling off, leaving skin of normal colour and patterning. When in doubt, dithranol 0.25% cream should be applied to previously treated areas for a further week or two.

Contraindications

Stop all dithranol treatments if there is moistness, discomfort, or soreness, or if there is more than a gradual spread of the psoriasis. Instead use yellow soft paraffin for a fortnight and then resume treatment sparingly as per the directions in 2 above but with the Dithrolan diluted with 4 parts of yellow soft paraffin, increasing the strength as tolerance develops. After the use of *local steroids*, first change to yellow soft paraffin for a fortnight. Then start dithranol 0.1% cream sparingly as per 2; alternatively the diluted Dithrolan may be used.

Insight

Early and complete clearance with dithranol or tar favourably alters the prognosis, whereas relapse usually follows the use of local steroids. The above physical treatment has greater lasting value when the patient is helped to understand and accept what precipitated the psoriasis. This insight is a vital factor in prognosis.

Chapter 4. Eczema, infantile eczema

While the physical changes in eczema and contact dermatitis are similar even microscopically, their history of onset and distribution are quite different. Eczema is mainly produced by internal causes and therefore the rashes tend to be symmetrical, whilst dermatitis tends to occur at the point of contact with the external physical factors. Dermatitis is described in Chapter 8.

The ability to cope in life depends upon inherited qualities, upbringing, training, intelligence and the degree of mental stability. The 'safety valve' for excessive pressure may appear as a psychiatric illness; alternatively the target organ may be the skin, as has been previously discussed. This pattern of expression is largely genetic; in eczema the skin is constitutionally prone to itching and to the eczematous changes to be described. These occur when the strain becomes unbearable, which is often the result of problems with interpersonal relationships:

> He had been an in-patient for 7 weeks. His extensive eczema improved initially but then relapsed. Each time a different area became excoriated and weeping. More significant was the fact that the relapses only took place on the morning of the expected ward round, and after his wife had visited him. The charge-nurse had already discovered that the patient was unhappy at home; the medical social worker's report indicated that little could be done. The consultant paid an unexpected visit; 'Your skin is quite clear—you can go home today'. 'But it's not ward-round morning, doctor; you can't do that!'

The eczemas can be acute, subacute or chronic. Characteristically there is *erythema* (reddening) and *oedema*, with discrete or groups of vesicles (small blisters) and *papules* (small elevations of the skin) giving the appearance of a uniform pin-head eruption. The vesicles weep and become secondarily infected and crusted. An intense itching or burning sensation causes the patient to rub and scratch, worsening the rash, and producing scaling and eventually *lichenification* (thickening) of the skin. Lichenified skin is much more prone to itch, and so a vicious circle becomes established.

Atopic eczema

Atopic eczema occurs in 3% of the population; 70% of the patients
have a positive family history. In atopy there is a genetic tendency to
allergic disorders; the patients suffer from eczema, asthma, hay-fever
and allergic rhinitis, either separately or in any combinations. There
may be an intolerance of certain proteins and foods such as eggs, fish,
cheese, orange juice and chocolate. This characteristic is often lost at
a later age, but then urticaria and migraine become more common
than in the rest of the population. In infancy there is occasionally a
history of eczema developing when cereals are introduced into the
diet, or of exacerbations taking place regularly after certain foods.
The IgE and IgG levels are raised. The patients tend to be emotionally
tense and unstable. Exacerbations occur at times of emotional upset,
infections, and exposure to allergens. In atopy there is also an increased incidence of geographical tongue, in which there is a patchy
migrating loss of the surface.

There is an associated congenital dry skin known as ichthyosis in
10% of patients with atopic eczema. It is present from birth to death
and does not vary with the eczema. Treatment is purely symptomatic
with emollient creams, but stirring 2 teaspoonfuls of deodorised ground
nut oil into the bath may be all that is needed.

The pathological changes are non-specific in eczema, but there are
three clinical pictures.

1   *Infantile*

The infantile type usually becomes apparent at about 2 months of
age, as erythema with small vesicles and crusts on an oedematous
surface. It mostly affects the face, especially the forehead and cheeks
(Plate 11). Also involved are the forearms, flexures, wrists and outer
surfaces of the legs, especially when the problem is extensive. This
form of eczema typically follows a remitting course, and usually clears
between 18 months and 4 years of age, commonly at 3–4 years.

There is an occasional non-atopic or seborrhoeic variety, which lasts
for a few weeks only and responds well to treatment with preparations
such as hydrocortisone with clioquinol.

2   *Childhood*

The childhood type usually starts after 4 years of age, but may follow
as a persistence of the infantile type. Papular or lichenified lesions

mostly occur on the flexural surfaces, and usually disappear by the age of 10–12 years.

3   *Adult*

The adult type may follow the infantile and childhood types, or may develop from puberty. The lesions are papular and lichenified; they affect the flexures (Fig. 16), neck, eyelids, face, wrists, and the back of the feet and hands. Chronicity will be common unless there is adequate physical treatment and psychological management.

Eczema herpeticum and vaccination

Eczema herpeticum and vaccination are rare vesicular, febrile illnesses which can result in death of the very young. They are caused by infection with the herpes or vaccinia viruses of a patient with eczema. It is

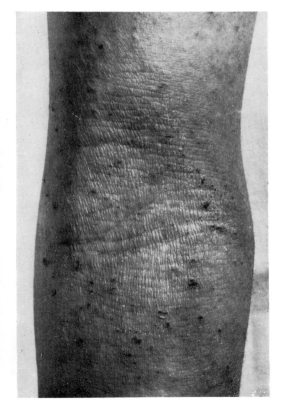

Fig. 16   Flexural eczema with lichenification.

therefore important for sufferers to avoid contact with the virus herpes simplex (cold sore), and they must never be vaccinated against small-pox; the rest of the inoculations may be given during a quiescent phase of the rash.

Discoid (nummular) eczema

Discoid (nummular) eczema is a presentation characterised by dry or weeping coin-shaped lesions (Plate 12). These typically occur in tense middle-aged people, but they can appear at any age and may follow an acute or chronic course. The sites affected are usually the calves, the back of the hands and forearms, and the front of the thighs. Associated flexural lesions may also be present.

Pompholyx

Pompholyx can be briefly described as eczema of thick skin. Sagograin vesicles appear on the palms and soles (Fig. 17), with irritation and later secondary infection. These episodes are usually seasonal and are thought to be due to inhaled allergens such as moulds. Eczema may

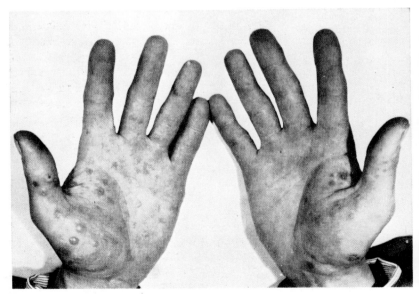

Fig. 17 Pompholyx showing profuse vesicles of thick skin.

be present elsewhere. Twice-daily 1 : 2000 soaks in potassium permanganate solution are useful to control any secondary infection, but otherwise treatment is the same as for eczema, to be described later.

Lichen simplex

Lichen simplex (lichenified eczema, neurodermatitis) consists of thickened papular and usually scaly lesions, which often become confluent. These mostly occur on the nape of the neck, the calves, and the outside of the forearms and ankles; in other words, on areas that are easy to scratch. The lesions are composed of extremely itchy and therefore lichenified skin, with a superimposed low-grade chronic infection from scratching. Sufferers often show signs of nervous tension, such as heavy smoking and drinking, nail biting, or hyperactivity —a sensitive inside and a sensitive outside:

'Why do I always relapse when I go to Leeds?' The eczema was scratched and lichenified, and affected the flexural aspects of the limbs, so aggravation from external factors was unlikely. The remark about Leeds spurred the doctor to question further, as he had trained there. 'Who lives at Leeds then?' 'My mother-in-law!'

Secondary absorption eczema

It is important to diagnose correctly any secondary absorption eczema in order for treatment to be effective. This can take place, for example, from an area of gravitational eczema around a leg ulcer, or from patches of contact dermatitis due to nickel fasteners. It usually affects the hands, forearms, neck and face. Patients suffering from eczema of the hands should always have their feet and legs carefully examined, and be specifically questioned about sensitivity to metals. Avoiding contact at the areas of primary absorption will help to clear the secondary eczema, together with the use of intermediate strength steroid creams.

Differential diagnosis

The differential diagnosis of eczema is based upon the character and progress of the lesions, plus a family history of the illness and associated conditions. Contact dermatitis has a different distribution and itches only in the presence of the external allergens. Seborrhoeic dermatitis does not occur on the limb flexures and typically itches less. Ringworm may mimic lichen simplex, but itches less and has a centre which is healing; also the edges of the fungal lesions show characteristic scaling. Anogenital pruritus may in fact be due to localised lichen simplex. In lichen planus the papules are polygonal, discrete and lilac coloured. All these conditions are described in greater detail in subsequent chapters. In psoriasis the lesions are more demarcated, and have a typical salmon pink colour and a different distribution.

Management

The management of eczema involves an understanding of its physical and psychological origins. Support and advice are needed, stressful situations being put into perspective wherever possible; insight is important. Nervous tension causes itching and therefore scratching which either produces or worsens the lesions. These then itch more intensely, and further scratching occurs with deterioration of the condition. This vicious circle must be broken before improvement can take place. Physical treatment must be given with confidence; patients should be instructed to make further topical applications to allay irritation, rather than to rub and scratch themselves.

Children require a quiet, stable, affectionate and balanced background; pampering or fussing over the child is often worse than neglect as it is liable to lead to flare-ups on demand, the child simply tearing at himself to get his own way! Communication between parent and child should be encouraged. The nurse can most readily do this by talking in front of the child; 'little pitchers have long ears!' This technique is similar to the doctor teaching the nurse in front of the patient, for the *patient's* benefit; conversely teaching the patient in front of the nurse for the *nurse's* benefit! This indirect approach makes communication so much easier, as it reduces the tension of being talked at. Finally don't forget that it is much less upsetting for children if their mother undresses them for examination out of sight of the nurse and doctor.

Regular meals and adequate periods of sleep are essential. Any known allergen should be avoided, such as certain foods for babies and sometimes moulds and pollens in children and adults. Foam mattresses and pillows will reduce any allergy to feathers. A stable surrounding temperature should be maintained and undressing in the cold avoided. Aggravating clothing such as woollens, straps and buckles, and local irritants such as detergents and cleansers should not be used; clothing should be well rinsed after washing, and soap replaced by oil or emulsifying ointment in personal hygiene.

All contact with water should be rigorously avoided in the acute phases of eczema. Once the rash comes under control, occasional washing of the non-affected sweaty areas can be permitted. Only when the lesions become quiescent can the affected areas be gently cleaned, and even then only with the emulsifying ointment.

Hospitalisation should be avoided unless the mother is admitted as well, certainly if the children are less than 2 years old; losing the person upon whom they most depend causes psychological upset which is important especially at this early age. Mother can be taught to undertake the child's treatment and have the joy of seeing the rash get better. Confidence and tranquillity must be restored, and opportunities made for discussing any of the mother's home problems. This can reduce family tension with great benefit to the child:

It was the expensive dictaphone that fascinated him. Mother was distraught trying to listen to the doctor's questions, pacify the 'hyperactive' child and prevent the room from being demolished! The doctor mused to himself on the saying that 'the sins of the parents are visited upon the children, even unto the third and fourth generations'. The consultation touched on what was upsetting the mother, and why she thought her marriage was breaking up. While the mother was engrossed, the child had become quiet, playing with some bobbins and a cocoa tin on the carpet. It was obvious that the mother had been projecting her own anxiety on to the child, who therefore felt insecure and sought attention. There was no need to change his treatment, but mother was also told to obtain a sedative to help her until the anxiety settled. General advice was accepted, and was ultimately effective. On enquiry 3 years later, the child's eczema was entirely clear and the mother really happy.

Large doses of sedatives are essential to reduce the level of mental activity and itching, in order to give the skin a chance to be cleared. Benzodiazepines such as diazepam (Valium) are commonly used, and must be given during the daytime as well as at night. In paediatric dermatology, promethazine (Phenergan elixir) is very useful as a sedative. Nails, of course, must be cut short in order to reduce their destructive power!

Antibiotics and antihistamines must not be used topically as the skin is easily sensitised. Unfortunately the skin is often already showing a superimposed contact dermatitis due to the handed-down and over-the-counter preparations already tried by the patient!

Staphylococcal infection can be superimposed on eczema to give an impetigenised rash. This is the usual cause of major exacerbations of the condition. Systemic antibiotics are then needed together with local steroids.

Topical steroids are the mainstay of treatment. The weaker preparations should always be used first, providing that the patient is continually improving. Rapid results can be obtained by applying the stronger steroid preparations in large quantities for a relatively short time. Weaker treatments are then needed to prevent therapeutic rebound and should be continued for at least 2 weeks after the skin looks and feels entirely normal. The local damage and systemic absorption should always be borne in mind with the long-term usage of strong steroids, especially when the surrounding skin is thin, as in the young. Occlusion under polythene may improve the effectiveness in the resistant areas. The polythene provides a barrier against physical attack from fingernails, but its main effect is to hydrate the keratin layer of the epidermis. This increases absorption of the steroid and enhances its effectiveness one hundred fold. Alexa ready-made polythene garments are of the correct shape, are easy to put on and can be worn for up to a day at a time. Secondary infection is the main contra-indication to polythene occlusion, as the hydrated keratin is readily invaded by organisms proliferating in the warm moist conditions. Watch for small erosions developing with indented outlines, similar to the shape of the islands in the West Indies (Fig. 27, page 60). Occlusion should then be stopped.

In the chronic lichenified stages, coal tar paste is an excellent preparation because of its antipruritic properties. The tar can also be impregnated with zinc paste into bandages. These are very effective in clearing severe lichenified eczema of the limbs. There is the antipruritic effect of the tar plus the physical protection from the bandage, both reducing scratching. Once the condition is nearly clear, used bandages can be reapplied just at night-time until the skin is perfect. Elastic adhesive plaster over coal tar paste bandages can be left in position for up to 2 weeks. Alternatively the outer covering can be made from two layers of tubular cotton gauze, or cotton bandage.

Intralesional hydrocortisone or triamcinalone injections can help the resolution of very lichenified eczema. Using a pressure jet (Dermojet) is less painful and quicker. Grenz rays or superficial X-rays may be used in older patients to reduce overactive areas. Their effect is only temporary, and they must therefore be used in conjunction with local and general therapy.

Severely affected patients may have to be admitted to hospital for treatment. The atmosphere of the ward is dependent upon confident nurses supported by experienced doctors. Some discipline in the ward is necessary, but this should be flexible and compassionate. Visitors should be encouraged except when ward rounds and medical examinations are taking place. Television can provide relaxing entertainment, but games involving exercise should be avoided as the activity spreads the ointments, and also causes sweating and irritation. A quiet area is needed so that patients are able to reflect on their problems and a more balanced perspective can then be achieved. The prognosis is improved if the patient remains in hospital until the rash has completely cleared, before returning home to any unresolved problems. It should not be forgotten that itching is increased by consumption of alcohol. Be enthusiastic with the therapy. Touch the patient with your fingers while examining, treating and talking to him. It restores confidence as society shuns a skin patient, just as it did the so-called lepers of the Middle Ages. With full psychological understanding and physical treatment the prognosis can be good, but otherwise relapses are common:

The old farmhouse was tucked away at the head of one of the lesser-known dales. The young doctor was taken there by the district nurse. There were two gates and then a stile where the road became a bridle-path for the final half mile. The patient was on her own, but she kept the house clean despite her 83 years of age and the primitive conditions in which she lived. Her eczema had started in patches within a week of her husband's sudden death. Life had become lonely and difficult, but she had managed on her own for 5 years. She now had difficulty in coping with her treatment as her rash had become generalised. Speedy admission to hospital was arranged, and the rash cleared. The patient had no insight, and continuous physical treatment was required to keep her comfortable at home until she died a year later.

Chapter 5. Prurigo, neurotic excoriations, artefacts, trichotillomania, alopecia areata, lichen planus

Prurigo

Prurigo is most easily described as a very localised lichenified eczema. The lesions are usually discrete and nodular (Fig. 18) but in the severer forms they can coalesce into sheets.

Treatment is virtually the same as for eczema, except that stronger measures are needed in the later stages due to the thickness of the lesions

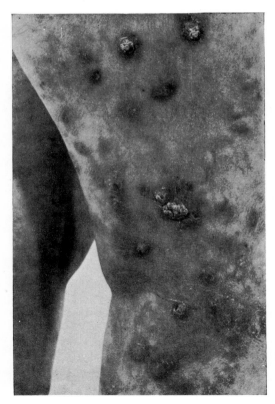

Fig. 18 Nodular prurigo showing discrete thickened lesions.

and the worse prognosis. Very strong steroid preparations are required but have to be applied accurately to prevent damage of the surrounding normal skin. Localisation is best effected by the use of elastic adhesive extension plaster, which also physically protects the skin from the patient's constant rubbing and scratching. Alternatively the steroid can be incorporated into a tape which is cut to the size of the lesion and then covered with the plaster. Coal tar paste bandages are not only antipruritic but also provide a physical barrier. As soon as there is improvement the adhesive plaster alone can be applied to the nodules. This is a very useful procedure as the plaster can be left in place for up to a fortnight at a time. In resistant lesions other measures such as intralesional steroid injections and Grenz rays may have to be used as in the treatment of lichenified eczema. Sedatives should also be given. Psychological support is needed as sufferers may alternate between prurigo and overt depressive illness. Without understanding this, treatment of either facet will simply result in a change of target organ.

Neurotic excoriations

Neurotic excoriations occur in patients who are under psychological stress. The obvious localised scratch marks and white scars from previous lesions occur round the neck, shoulders (Figs. 19, 20) and limbs, but also at any other site where the patient can scratch. The palatal and corneal reflexes are often reduced or absent. There may be a glint in the patient's eye which in effect says 'This is the way I express myself, and I dare you to stop me!'

Management is difficult but psychotherapy can be helpful if given early. It is all too easy in the pressures of modern medical life to think of people as 'cases' and forget that they are also patients. Neurotics especially are in need of understanding. Local treatment is with fairly strong antipruritics such as menthol 1.5% with phenol 2% in calamine lotion. Patients should be instructed to apply this whenever they feel any irritation rather than to attack themselves. Safe sedatives such as the benzodiazepines should be used, as they are not very effective as suicidal agents.

Artefacts

Artefacts give the appearance of having been produced by an external physical agent. They should be suspected whenever there are straight, bizarre or angular markings (Fig. 21) or lesions which do not follow the natural contours of the body. They are solely produced or per-petuated by subconscious actions by the patient; in malingering the

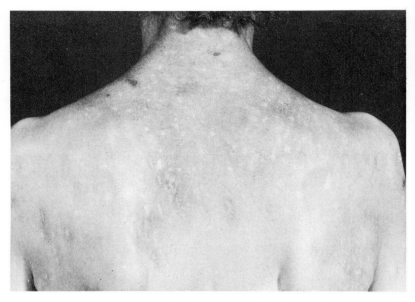

Fig. 19   Neurotic excoriations showing two recent lesions and many scars from previous ones.

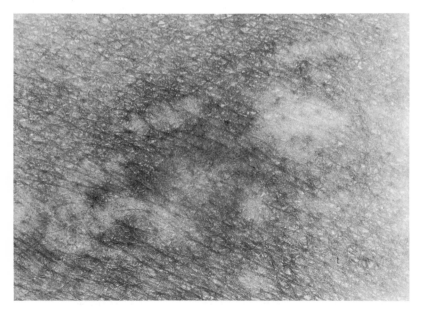

Fig. 20   Neurotic excoriations, a closer view of the scars.

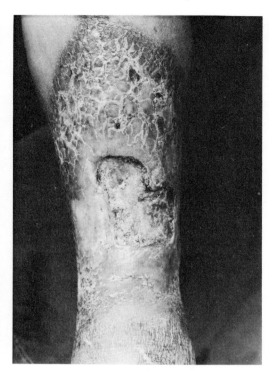

Fig. 21 Longstanding artefact ulcer of leg showing straight edges.

actions are conscious. The sites must be accessible, are usually multiple, and in the more intelligent may mimic a recognised skin lesion. The way that they are produced varies from chemicals, veterinary plasters, pressure necrosis from elastic bands, to picking and scratching with the fingernails and other implements.

Artefacts are much commoner in females, especially in the 20–30 age group. Emotional factors are always present, and the diagnosis can often be suspected from the patient's nature and manner of speaking; there may be hysterical behaviour, overemphasis, or disassóciated remarks:

> She was in bed, but her expression was serene. A band of painful ulcers had suddenly developed all round the lower part of the left leg. To the question, 'How did you produce them?' came the disassociated reply, 'My husband's an invalid and I have to take in visitors. I am 56.' Healing in hospital was uneventful but the pain persisted. An X-ray showed nipping of the tibia and fibula like a belt round 2 pulleys. Despite her protestations that no encircling band could be present, it was agreed to operate. The orthopaedic surgeon was able to remove what he expected to find—an elastic band! (Figs. 22, 23.)

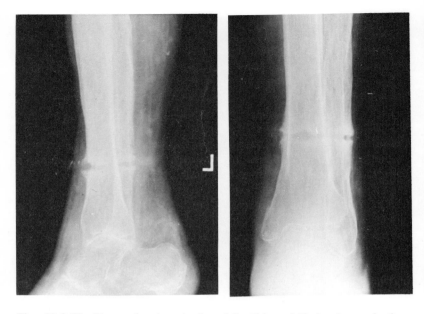

Figs. 22 & 23   X-rays showing nipping of the tibia and fibula—by an elastic band.

The lesions are outward signs of psychological illness. The patient must be given support and understanding while the rash gets better. Safe sedatives should again be used. Crystal violet 0.25% in aqueous cream is a useful local treatment which aids healing and provides evidence of its use; it is messy enough to discourage the production of further lesions, and its colour gives the patient a visible excuse for getting better. Early therapy will produce a better prognosis. Referral to a psychiatrist is mandatory for those who do not improve.

Occlusive dressings give the best protection and enable natural healing. Marking of the bandages is essential to show that they have not been disturbed, but even this is not 100% foolproof; it is surprising what damage a knitting needle can do if pushed under the dressings! Only Plaster of Paris or polyurethane cast bandages (Bayercast) give secure protection, and are invaluable for out-patients. They also have the advantage of being a physical decoy from which the patients can obtain the desired attention and support from their friends and relations! The appearance of fresh lesions above or below an occlusive dressing is not only diagnostic of artefact but is also an indication that the patient's problems have not been solved.

Trichotillomania

Trichotillomania is due to subconscious removal or breaking of hair, producing areas of relatively bald scalp covered by normal, but broken, ends of hair. Children usually grow out of this problem but it is best to find the cause and give advice accordingly. Asking the parent 'how does he produce them' is the quickest way of establishing rapport. Adults usually need psychotherapy of varying degree. Trichotillomania and artefacts are both rare. They have been included in this chapter as examples of external manifestations of psychological problems where the mode of production of the lesions is known. The same cannot yet be said of alopecia areata and lichen planus where an autoimmune cause is probable, although psychological factors are still important.

Alopecia areata

Alopecia areata may follow ordeals, domestic upsets or bereavements. Characteristically there are single or multiple areas of well-defined round or oval patches of hair loss (Fig. 24). These may coalesce to involve the whole scalp (alopecia totalis) and even the entire body (alopecia universalis). The onset may be insidious, or sudden and dramatic. The diagnostic features are smooth areas which are neither scaling nor scarred, and the presence of 'exclamation mark' hairs; the last mentioned are short club-shaped hair stumps whose broken ends are thicker than their bases.

The condition is non-infective, affecting both sexes equally and occurring at any age but more commonly in childhood. There is a family history of the condition in about 20% of sufferers and also an association with diabetes and vitiligo. Any prior stress should be identified and discussed. Anxiety will result in overattention in the form of brushing and combing, thus removing the surrounding loose hairs and apparently worsening the condition. These hairs are in the resting phase, as described on page 207. Treatment with bland applications and confidence is the rule, with special attention to good health which in itself takes the mind off the condition. Tonics and iron are frequently used along with topical steroid creams and lotions. However their value may only be psychological. Reactions produced by the local application of dinitrochlorbenzene or cantharides may be effective in patients who have not done well.

In most cases the hair regrows. As resolution starts the 'exclamation marks' disappear and are replaced by a thin covering of 'down'. The

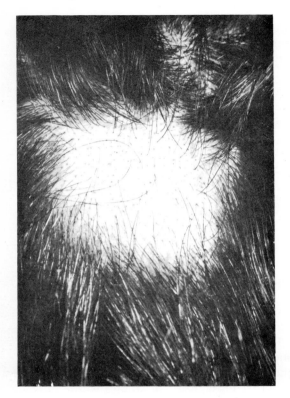

Fig. 24 Alopecia areata showing some '!' mark hairs.

surrounding hair then thickens up and becomes firmer. Ringworm, mentioned on page 121, may mimic alopecia areata but close examination will reveal no 'exclamation marks', and the diagnosis can be confirmed by a Wood's lamp or by microscopy and culture. In psoriasis and seborrhoea there is an abnormal scalp surface with no broken hairs.

Diffuse alopecia

Diffuse alopecia occurs within 2 months of a severe illness such as meningitis or stress and may last for up to 2 years. It may also occur during hormonal changes such as in myxoedema, following delivery, the menopause, or after stopping the contraceptive pill. Alopecia is also produced by cytotoxic drugs and radiation from a direct physical action on the hair follicles.

The most common form of alopecia (95%) is 'male pattern' baldness which is a familial condition. It also is worsened by physical or psychological illness. The condition mainly affects men and is characterised by a recession of the hairline from the fronto-parietal regions. Although a lot of money is spent on remedies no treatment has ever been proved to be effective. Hair transplants are considered on page 185.

Wigs can help all alopecia sufferers and give the hair underneath a chance to recover by preventing overattention. Best quality made-to-measure, man-made fibre wigs are suitable for short-term problems. They have an advantage over hair wigs in that they are cheaper and can be washed. Wigs must look good to give the patients confidence and take their mind off the emotionally upsetting sight that confronts them from each mirror they pass.

'A woman's crowning glory is her hair' (Goldsmith):

> She was 40 and had a diffuse alopecia. It was noticeable that she presented much of the rest of her anatomy for examination! Patients tell their own stories in many different ways—by their movements, posture, expression, or even how they flutter their eyelids! It was the family doctor who knew the answer to the problem—her diabetic husband was becoming impotent.

Lichen planus

Lichen planus is rare in childhood, occurs in women more than men, and usually follows a self-limiting course of between 6 and 18 months. It may also be related to shock or stress:

> The roof had caved in when he had been checking equipment at the coal face. He had heard the rockfall when the lights went out. He inspected it with his hand-lamp, but there was no escape. There is a great comradeship in the mines and rescue teams work fast. Even so it was 2 days before he reached the surface; by then he was covered by lichen planus.

Lichen planus is composed of small, flat-topped, shiny, lilac-coloured polygonal papules (Plate 13), sometimes showing dimpled centres and fine striae (Wickham's). The degree of itching is variable. The areas commonly affected are the wrists, forearms, inner thighs and genitals, with or without trunk involvement. It may also occur as a Koebner phenomenon at actual points of injury. Vesicles and bullae are uncommon. If the lesions fuse they may mimic psoriasis.

Lesions in the mouth may occur even without those on the skin, presenting as striae of the buccal mucosa (Plate 14). These lines are composed of white papules, giving a lace-curtain effect. The nails may also be involved to a varying degree, from accentuated longitudinal ridges to complete and permanent loss of the whole nail. The scalp is seldom affected, but when it does occur the hair loss is permanent, as the lesions result in the destruction of the hair follicles. Malignancy does occur following persistent lichen planus of the mouth, but is rare.

Treatment is the same as that described for longstanding eczema, from page 46, except that washing the skin is not restricted. Local steroids are useful as antipruritics. Strong ones are needed for thick lesions, sometimes with the addition of polythene occlusion. Extensive cases benefit from tapering courses of systemic steroids. Sedatives are needed to reduce tension, allay irritation and ensure sleep. Lichen planus heals leaving a brown colour in the 'white' races and extra pigmentation in those whose skin is already dark. Treatment should only cease when the lesions have entirely lost their substance. The pigment will then disappear a few months afterwards. Mouth lesions should first be treated with hydrocortisone hemisuccinate (Corlan) pellets. Resistant areas may need the use of equal quantities of a very strong local steroid ointment mixed with triamcinalone in orabase. Carbolic solution 2% should also be used as a mouth wash if there is soreness.

Management is all important:

> She lived at one end of her mother-in-law's farmhouse and was treated like a servant. She had been promised a house of her own by her husband since their marriage 17 years before; but he was dominated by his mother and submitted to her view that there was plenty of room in the existing building. She was now 36. The subject was again brought up, but this time she did the talking. There was a family row. Three days later she was covered with lichen planus. At consultation the family doctor's treatment could not be improved upon, so no change was advised. There were tears as soon as her home circumstances were discussed, but she was happier when she left, although she realised there was little chance of domestic change. The next consultation was 6 weeks later. All that remained of the rash was the normal residual pigmentation that follows the disorder. Only reassurance was needed that it would take about 2 months for this to disappear entirely.

Chapter 6. Seborrhoeic dermatitis, acne, rosacea, anogenital pruritus

Patients suffering from the conditions included in this chapter usually have the hereditary tendency to seborrhoea, which is an excessive production of sebum; this is produced by sebaceous glands to protect, grease and maintain the surface of the skin. Its production is under the hormonal control of the androgens, so seborrhoea is usually present around puberty and for a few years afterwards. The skin is then more readily affected by normal commensal organisms whose overgrowth causes a sensitising dermatitis. This is seen more frequently in association with psychological pressure, and together with rubbing and scratching is responsible for the eczematisation. The endogenous and exogenous causes have led to the condition being variously called *seborrhoeic eczema* or *seborrhoeic dermatitis*. As candida and other low-grade infections can be demonstrated bacteriologically, the term *dermatitis* is more commonly used and will be adopted here.

Seborrhoeic dermatitis

Seborrhoeic dermatitis affects areas which are rich in sebaceous glands, namely the nose, central face, scalp (Fig. 25), and to a lesser extent the upper chest and back. It also affects surfaces in apposition where there is friction and moistness, and is known as intertrigo or sweat rash. It is therefore found in the axillae, groins, umbilicus, submammary and other folds in obese patients. The hair is usually greasy. The scalp, eyelids, ears, beard area and corners of the mouth may all be affected.

The condition has a gradual onset and may run an acute, subacute or chronic inflammatory course. On skin and scalp the scales are grey or dirty yellow in colour and may be either dry or greasy. The macules or papules are up to 1 cm in diameter; when extensive they may become confluent, fissured, moist and infected with crusts.

The general treatment of seborrhoeic disorders is to reduce the quantity of low-grade infection. The inherited tendency cannot be changed, but much can be done to alleviate the condition. Dealing

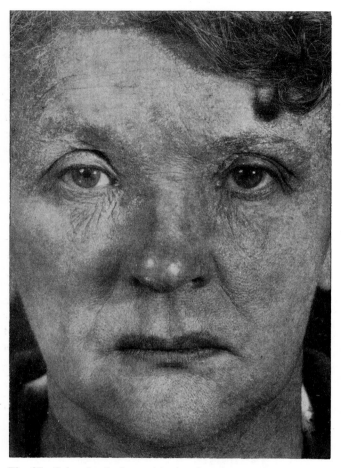

Fig. 25 Seborrhoeic dermatitis showing characteristic superficial scaling which also involved the scalp.

with any psychological problem is important and this is discussed at the end of the section. Correction of diet is helpful; sufferers should reduce their consumption of carbohydrate and solid fat, and instead take more undercooked vegetables, salads, fruits and proteins.

The quantity of low-grade infection can be reduced by regular bathing or washing, but eroded rashes can be aggravated by water. Most seborrhoeic eruptions benefit from a sulphur and salicylic acid (3%) ointment BP which is cheap but greasy. Preparations such as econazole are more effective and are mentioned where the site of the infection is being described.

Miliaria rubra

Prickly heat, also known as *miliaria rubra*, should not be confused with a diffuse seborrhoeic pustular folliculitis. It is an acute rash of minute inflammatory papules and vesicles at the orifices of the sweat glands, common amongst 'white' races in the tropics. It is due to maceration causing swelling of the horny cells round the ducts. Polythene occlusion can also cause it. Management includes avoiding sweating from exertion, and friction from clothing whenever possible. Fans are helpful, but air-conditioning is the most effective treatment. Calamine lotion should be applied and large doses of ascorbic acid taken.

Intertrigo

In intertrigo the areas are red, moist and confluent and affect right up into and including the flexure surfaces. Napkin (diaper) dermatitis may look very similar except that the actual flexures are not involved, as they do not come into contact with the sodden, irritant nappy (Fig. 26). Apart from avoiding this irritation, the treatment of napkin dermatitis is the same as intertrigo and will now be discussed. The irritation of wet nappies is due mainly to the maceration, the secondary infection and the effect of the ammonia from the stale urine. Frequent changing of nappies is therefore needed, and it is best to apply them only as a skirt; plastic pants are forbidden. After each change, local treatment such as a silicone barrier cream, zinc and castor oil cream, or benzalkonium chloride with cetrimide cream should be applied. The preparations mentioned in the next paragraph are stronger but may be needed if the condition fails to respond.

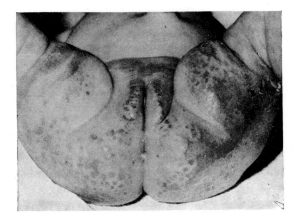

Fig. 26 Napkin dermatitis with characteristic sparing of the creases.

The treatment of intertrigo should be based on keeping the areas cool and dry with either talcum powder or gauze, and also reducing secondary infection. A variety of antiseptics may be used, the cheapest being crystal violet 0.5% in calamine lotion; econazole cream is cleaner and equally effective. Hydrocortisone cream with miconazole or clioquinol is often recommended; the weak steroid improves the dermatitis and therefore hastens progress. Polynoxylin powder is effective when there is Gram-negative infection, as are soaks with silver nitrate 0.5% in water, applied on gauze every 3 hours and moistened twice at night (Fig. 27).

Pyogenic infection persists where there are cracks at the apex of an area of intertrigo or fissures behind the ears; frequent applications of either the crystal violet or silver nitrate are quickly effective. If only daily treatment is possible, the lotion should be allowed to dry and then sealed in position with an acrylic resin spray.

Antibiotics taken internally alter the body's normal bacteriological flora; they kill off the organisms that are sensitive and allow an overgrowth of those that are resistant. *Candida* is resistant and can be a complication of antibiotic therapy, and is seen dermatologically as thrush in the mouth or as an intertrigo. Overgrowth of resistant Gram-

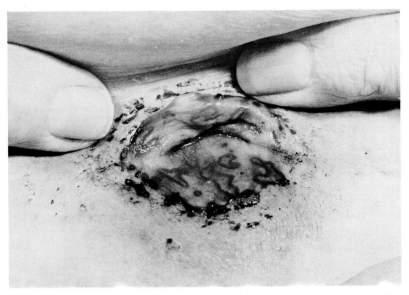

Fig. 27   Gram-negative erosions of the umbilicus showing typical outlines like the islands of the West Indies. Pseudomonas was grown on culture.

negative and other infections are also encountered. Diabetes is another cause of intertrigo due to *Candida*, and the urine should always be tested when an infected rash is diagnosed.

Mention should be made of an intertrigenous condition called *angular stomatitis*. The gums may recede following the wearing of false teeth; this causes the jaws to come close together and produces a fold at the angles of the mouth with an extension of the moist areas. Dentures that are too shallow have the same effect. Secondary invaders, usually *Candida*, cause the localised dermatitis. Vitamin B and iron deficiency should first be excluded, and the bite adjusted by redesigning the dentures and attention paid to their hygiene. Locally miconazole with hydrocortisone cream (Daktacort) should be applied every few hours for a fortnight after the condition has cleared.

Seborrhoeic blepharitis

Seborrhoeic blepharitis (of the eyelids) should not be treated with chemicals which might irritate the eye. Unfortunately topical antibiotics have to be used; these include oxytetracycline or chlortetracycline which do not normally sensitise the skin. Adding hydrocortisone 1% is again beneficial.

When there is infection of the beard (sycosis), strong preparations are needed such as clioquinol with fluorandrenolone cream (Haelan C), or miconazole with hydrocortisone cream. Electric razors are less traumatic, and a change in shaving habit is often beneficial. Systemic antibiotics may be required in addition, as with any seborrhoeic problems that do not respond to local treatments. They should be given in reduced dosage but over a longer period, as will be described for acne.

Pityriasis capitis

Pityriasis capitis (dandruff) may clear through using shampoos such as cetrimide or selenium disulphide once or twice weekly. Clotrimazole or betamethasone alcoholic scalp applications are more effective. These should be applied once daily, in conjunction with the shampooing once or twice a week as mentioned above. It is best to continue with a medicated shampoo such as Wright's Coal Tar to prevent relapse. Care of the normal scalp is discussed on page 207.

Otitis externa

Otitis externa has two main causes. The low-grade infection causes irritation, weeping and oedema of the meatal orifice; the irritation can also be produced by psychomatic factors. Instead of asking patients, 'Do you rub or scratch your ears?' it is far more effective to get straight to the point by saying, 'What do you use to scratch inside your ears?!' Local treatment is best with spirit-based preparations, even though there may be a little initial stinging. Betamethasone alcoholic application used as drops twice daily gives the quickest results; the addition of phenoxyethanol 2% and crystal violet 0.25% may be required if infection persists. Clotrimazole alcoholic solution is nearly as effective. Silver nitrate 0.25% in 70% spirit is best for the treatment of *Pseudomonas aeruginosa*. Debris should be removed when possible as it is irritant and harbours secondary infection. This can be carried out by the ENT team using a special hook. Alternatively the ear can be syringed, but it must be realised that the water from this procedure will temporarily delay progress. Wax in the ears should be softened by daily applications of vegetable oil for 3 days before the syringing is carried out. Patients of course should be warned to keep water out of the ears while washing; they must not go swimming for a fortnight after the ears have healed.

Treatment

Numerous local applications have already been suggested for the treatment of seborrhoeic infections in various parts of the body, and it is sometimes difficult to avoid poly-prescribing! It is equally important to treat the patient as a whole individual and not just the affected areas of the skin. Sufferers are often depressed, resentful and anxious, with inadequate personalities. They should be helped with their problems, sedated and allowed to rest. Most attacks settle within 7 weeks, but upsets may cause relapse or persistence for much longer unless full psychological understanding is obtained.

'Why do I live under so much tension?' He was 32 and had come about his dandruff, which always worsened at the year-end when his profits were assessed. His business was a tremendous financial achievement, but he could not understand why it mattered so much to him. 'Does your wife love you?' He looked really startled, but after a long pause said, 'Thank you for asking me; I know now why I needed the achievement I didn't get at home—but why didn't I see all this before?'
The consultant explained, 'It is because we have no insight that we do not see problems we do not want to face. Nature has shown that evolution is effective only when the ability to cooperate with one's fellows and environment is well developed. For physical survival some self-interest is obviously necessary, but when this is carried into the social field, and especially when it is overemphasised, it inevitably leads

to frustration and stress. This self-centred activity at any level causes conflict inwardly and outwardly, and a failure to face up to life as it really is. Self-deception to bolster oneself up then follows and this produces further stress. We can only see ourselves as we really are as a reflection; by watching how we react to our environment, that is to people, ideas and things. But it is much easier to explain all this than carry it out oneself. When we sat our competitive examinations, all our collars were covered with dandruff!'

Acne vulgaris

Acne vulgaris (or 'teenage spots') is a common association of the seborrhoeic skin. Acne usually develops after puberty and disappears by 30 years of age. It is due to an abnormal sensitivity to the slight increase in androgens and is therefore absent in eunuchs. The condition is worse in damp, dull climates, in winter, and in times of stress such as examinations or before menstrual periods. Acne patients are probably more upset by their rash than any other group in dermatology. Embarrassment may occur and lead to self-consciousness, shyness and restriction in the normal enjoyment of life.

The condition is characterised by comedones (blackheads) which are due to sebum in the glands being held back by horny plugs of keratinised protein (Fig. 28). The triglycerides in the sebum become altered by the commensal organisms into irritant fatty acids. These cause surrounding chronic inflammation and the formation of pustules, cysts and small abscesses. It is a gradual process with an insidious onset, affecting the face, chest, back and the neck, and often associated with greasy skin and dandruff. If left untreated, permanent scarring will occur.

Treatment

Persistence is the mainstay in the treatment of acne. It is likely that it is the caring and enthusiasm that works in the initial stages, as it takes at least a month for physical treatment to start being effective. The skin should be thoroughly cleaned each evening with soap and warm water. A preparation such as one containing benzoyl peroxide 5% in a gel base should be carefully applied in increasing quantities each evening, providing no soreness or scaling develops.

Ultraviolet light from conventional mercury vapour lamps is also useful as it causes scaling. Exposure to winds, weather and natural sunlight is also beneficial. However, sweating should be avoided wherever possible, along with physical trauma to the skin such as the

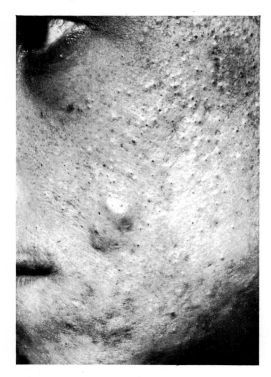

Fig. 28 Acne vulgaris
showing many
blackheads and a few
cystic lesions.

rubbing of a collar or coat. Once a week, the blackheads should be
expressed with a comedone extractor or hair grip. Pustules must be
left severely alone to minimise scarring.

Intralesional triamcinalone using the dermojet may prove useful in
the treatment of cysts. Treatment with a carbon dioxide stick or slush,
described on page 184, is effective. Tetracycline, oxytetracycline or
erythromycin 250 mg twice daily should be taken for several months,
and during this period at least 2 cartons of natural yoghurt a week
should be consumed to replenish the gut with non-pathogenic bacteria.
The antibiotic appears to work by reducing the number of commensal
organisms in the skin lesions. The tetracyclines are absorbed better if
taken with water half an hour before meals. Hormones may help young
girls with a persisting rash; the contraceptive pill can be used for a
short period in up to double standard dose, but it must contain a
non-androgenic progestogen.

A diet high in cooked and uncooked vegetables is recommended,
along with plenty of salads and fruit. Solid fats should be rationed as
their ingestion probably affects the composition of sebum; butter and

lard should be replaced by a soft margarine made from soya or corn oil. Cocoa, sugar, chocolate and fatty meat should be avoided. With proper management, a 90% cure should be expected but may take several months.

Acne variants

Acne conglobata (cystic acne) is a rare variant resulting in abscesses, sinuses and scars, and may also involve the apocrine glands of the axillae, buttocks and perineum. Surgical removal of the affected areas is sometimes necessary.

Acne keloid is a chronic staphylococcal infection of hair follicles on the back of the neck, causing an abnormal keloid response. The condition is more common in Negroes. Clioquinol or sodium fucidate with an intermediate strength steroid are useful topical preparations. Once the keloid has formed, intralesional triamcinalone or plastic surgery may be required.

Occupational acne involves contact with oils, waxes and chemicals, especially some of the chlorinated hydrocarbons, and usually affects the limbs of people working with thin mineral oils. Iatrogenic acne can follow the ingestion of iodides, bromides, ACTH and some oral steroids.

Infantile acne usually occurs in male babies within the first year. Local treatment is usually effective, but if antibiotics are needed, erythromycin must be used as the tetracyclines stain and damage the developing teeth.

Acne excoria is a variant which involves the compulsive picking of acne lesions on the face, and usually occurs in females with an obsessional neurosis. The patients tend to be tense and anxious, often with demanding or rigid parents.

Rosacea

Rosacea is another condition with increased seborrhoeic activity. Pustular or non-follicular papular chronic inflammatory lesions are present on the face, especially on those areas that the circus clown paints red! There is also a persisting blush or erythema, with resulting permanent dilatation of the blood vessels (telangiectasia). It occurs more often in females, usually over 30 years of age and especially around the menopause. It involves an unstable vasomotor system, and is influenced particularly by emotional upsets or hormonal changes.

Severe cases result in papules and acneform pustules on the erythematous base (Plate 15), and the eyes may become involved as keratitis and corneal ulcers develop. The sebaceous glands of the nose may undergo excessive hypertrophy as a rhinophyma, which may even require plastic surgery.

Diagnosis and treatment

The differential diagnosis of rosacea is mainly acne vulgaris which has comedones, and lupus erythematosus in which the rash is not acneform in nature. Excessive alcohol, spices, sunlight and prolonged exposure to strong winds are included in the physical causes. These should be avoided along with excessive washing, and treatment should be with bland preparations or cold creams. Potent corticosteroids should be avoided (Plate 16) as they will increase the telangiectasia and prematurely age the skin. Sulphur 1% in calamine lotion or a 2% sulphur and salicylic acid cream are effective for the treatment of papules and pustules. A low dosage of a tetracycline should again be used for long periods until the skin is clear. This is the best treatment for any residual erythema.

Ladies should use non-sensitising cosmetics to disguise the rash while they regain confidence in themselves and to prevent secondary worry from the rash. Psychotherapy is important; there should be support and investigation of any emotional factors, together with reassurance and sedation. Occasionally the rash may be due to guilt:

> Her rosacea had resisted treatment, so the young consultant arranged for his 35-year-old patient to be seen by his principal teacher. Some changes in treatment were suggested but none were effective. It was years later that her family doctor phoned up specially, 'Yes, it was the patient who didn't seem to mind that her husband was often away at sea. There had been no change in her rash, but a domestic crisis developed when he was given a job near home. Rather than face life without her lover, she had committed suicide.'

Anogenital pruritus

Anogenital pruritus includes pruritus ani, pruritus scroti, pruritus vulvae, and balanitis. These conditions are mainly caused in two ways: firstly by low-grade infection as in seborrhoeic dermatitis, and secondly by psychological stress producing the vicious circle of itching, scratching and eczematisation exactly as described for lichenified eczema. Both causes may be present at the same time. For simplicity they will be discussed separately.

Intertrigo and balanitis caused by diabetes or antibiotic therapy are all pruritic. Haemorrhoids (piles), trichomonas, threadworms, pubic lice, candida and ringworm can all be extremely irritant, and the correct diagnosis must always be made before appropriate treatment is commenced. Menopausal and senile atrophy can also cause pruritus. Allergy to rubber sheaths, spermicidal creams or local applications of the benzocaine type may cause an irritant contact dermatitis. Anogenital pruritus due to psychological stress is usually a local manifestation of lichenified eczema. There may be anxiety, fear of pregnancy, revulsion to intercourse, or the condition may be due to the subconscious rejection of marital responsibility. When the areas involved have sexual significance, 'too much, too little or the wrong sort', is a quip based on some foundation! Flexural psoriasis is a similar but less common presentation:

> Although only 37 years old she appeared to be at least 50, with wrinkled brow and drooped shoulders. Her flexural psoriasis of the vulval region (Plate 3) developed shortly after the birth of her thirteenth child. She looked worn out. The rash was so sore that intercourse was impossible. She was terrified of having further children, but her religion forbade the use of contraceptive methods. Repeated attempts in hospital failed to clear her condition until she developed an infected uterus which had to be removed. Conception was then impossible, and the psoriasis quickly cleared within a fortnight using only the weak dithranol ointment.

It is a pity from the diagnostic point of view that particular emotional problems do not always affect particular sites on the skin. The face however may be involved when there is embarrassment, feelings of guilt, or when the 'flag of distress is being shown' (Plate 1), as in rosacea, psoriasis or seborrhoeic dermatitis. The palms and soles certainly can be areas of emotional expression, the upset being manifested as psoriasis, eczema or pompholyx.

There are many facets to human relationship, and it is only by caring and with tenderness that they can be unravelled. This certainly applies to any psychological cause of anogenital pruritus. Small doses of sedatives or antihistamines are helpful. Depression should be treated, if present, as the itch threshold is lowered in this disorder.

Testing the patient's urine for sugar is mandatory. A vaginal swab and a skin scraping should be taken for microscopy and culture. These tests are required to supplement the history and physical examination. After making the diagnosis, the appropriate preparation can be applied. This would include the use of nystatin or econazole pessaries and creams for candida, fungus or erythrasma infections. Trichomonas should be treated with di-iodohydroxyquinoline (Floraquin) pessaries, supplemented with oral metronidazole (Flagyl), which should also be given to the partner.

Soothing baths are beneficial, such as potassium permanganate 1:8000, but high temperatures should be avoided as they cause sweating and further itching. Miconazole with hydrocortisone has the advantage of being effective against yeast, fungi and low-grade infection while the hydrocortisone is a safe antipruritic. It should not be forgotten however that commonsense advice, such as gently sponging the anal region after defecating, or advising marital partners may be more effective than pills and potions:

She had been a widow for many years, and now had married someone younger than herself. The mild vulvitis responded to compound lead lotion, but she still felt sore after intercourse. On enquiry as to whether she was readjusting to married life again, she said, 'Yes, I'm so happy—but he's very strong.'

Doctors and nurses not only have to give simple advice at times to marital partners, but have to know that KY lubricant jelly is not only of use for medical examinations!

Chapter 7. Urticaria and drug eruptions

Urticaria

Urticaria is a condition consisting of transient erythematous weals, otherwise known as 'hives' or 'nettle rash' (Fig. 29). There is a pricking or itching sensation which may be severe. It can be acute, chronic or recurrent, but the lesions leave no permanent trace. Females are affected more often than males, and at any age, but more often in the 30–40 age group.

Each lesion appears suddenly and persists for between 1 and 48 hours. Attacks last from a few days to a few weeks in the acute stages

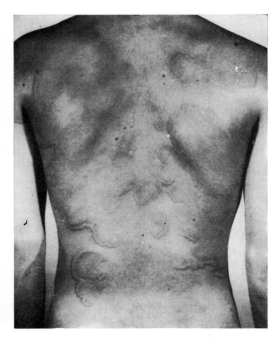

Fig 29. Acute urticaria with erythematous and annular lesions.

and in chronic urticaria they can recur for many years. The lesions are of variable size and may coalesce. The common sites affected are the arms, legs, thighs and waist. In the acute stage there may be slight pyrexia, and occasionally joint effusions.

A typical feature which helps to make the diagnosis is that each individual lesion does not last for more than 48 hours, nor is there any subsequent scaling of the skin as seen in dermatitis. Also the onset of the rash is usually within 2 hours as compared with over 12 hours in dermatitis.

The lesions are produced by certain substances released from the mast cells in the skin, which include histamine and serotonin. Physical agents such as heat, cold or pressure can also cause this release from the cells. The stinging nettle injects similar chemicals which produce an identical rash by direct action on the blood vessels.

Angioneurotic oedema (giant urticaria) is a more severe, rare and potentially dangerous form of urticaria. The lesions are bigger, more subcutaneous and cover larger and more important areas; eyelid involvement may completely close the eyes, lip and tongue involvement may prevent eating and laryngeal involvement may even stop breathing. The condition has a strong familial component.

Many of the acute urticarias are allergic in origin, due to hypersensitivity reactions. The allergens vary; the majority are drug induced, and are dealt with later in this chapter. It must be remembered that drugs include over-the-counter preparations consumed by all of us from time to time. Foods can cause urticaria, commonly shellfish, lobster, pork, nuts, and egg proteins. Food preservatives or the dyes added to foods and medicinal tablets can also be responsible. Even the quinine in tonic water can cause it!

A large proportion of the chronic urticarias have a psychogenic component, usually being associated with resentment, emotional conflict or anxiety neurosis; the life situation appears unjust and the patient is completely unable to do anything about it.

Management

Management of the urticarias includes identification and avoidance of any causative factor. Close attention to detail is required with regard to the times of ingestion and onset of the rash. Even the surgeon and physician who do not believe in psychiatry always teach that a full history is always necessary; during consultation, the patients themselves may gain understanding into any psychological origins of their rash:

The young locum had much scientific knowledge and intellect, but he was not convinced that rashes could be produced by stress and much preferred to deny its existence. He was an expert in allergic and immune problems. Why a 35-year-old patient with chronic urticaria should be sent for skin testing was beyond him; one diagnosed the rare but obvious allergens from the history, whereas here was one of the many cases where no cause would be found. 'When did your rash start?' 'When my husband left me.' 'Yes, but when? What year was that?' 'Just before the rash appeared.' By now the patient was crying. Antihistamines were prescribed, but before she left she confided to sister, 'I thought that I had got over being on my own. I don't need these pills, thank you.'

Cold compresses, tepid baths, calamine, and steroid lotions or creams give symptomatic relief. Antihistamines are the treatment of choice; they should be given in large enough doses to completely suppress the condition. In chronic urticaria the dosage should be reduced gradually and only after the skin has been clear for a full month. In acute cases oral steroids may also be needed, or even subcutaneous adrenaline (0.5–1.0 ml of 1:1000 solution) in an emergency; certain patients may need to carry the injection for self-administration, which can be life-saving.

Identification of an allergen may then be extremely important. This can be undertaken by carrying out an elimination diet of water and glucose, with foodstuffs being added one at a time at intervals of not less than 48 hours. The diet is time-consuming and patients can sometimes do their own investigations if they keep a very careful diary record of what they eat and how their skin varies. However, only a few positive results are obtained in those who suffer from the chronic form of urticaria. Why this is so is not clear. Is it because the development of a mild reaction to an allergen depends partly on the psychological state of the individual? This has certainly been observed in other conditions which also have the familial component, such as hay fever:

If the consultant started sneezing on the ward round, the staff always knew that a treatment error had been made. The incubation time was within minutes, the incident often being amusing enough to defuse the situation! It only happened in the hay-fever season. The consultant, who was then single-handed, had observed that the rush of completing his work before a holiday always worsened his hay fever, making the drive north to the Black Cuillins of Skye unpleasant. The relaxation of rock-climbing soon meant that the antihistamines could be stopped. During the journey back south, the smell of hay could actually be enjoyed. What was fascinating was that it was only necessary to resort to the use of antihistamines after returning to the stress of administrative work.

Drug eruptions

Drug eruptions are commonly urticarial in form and, as already described, are due to an acquired sensitisation.

Allergic reactions to drugs tend to run in families and can occur at any age. They appear in the more anxious types, and females tend to be affected more often than males. Antibiotics, hypnotics and tranquillisers are the worst offenders, sensitisation occurring following previous exposure to that drug or a chemically related substance; for example, if a patient is sensitive to penicillin then other penicillin-based antibiotics will cause a drug eruption. This is known as cross-sensitivity. A generalised histamine release may result in serum sickness, or even anaphylaxis, and details of the mechanisms involved are discussed at the beginning of Chapter 9.

The increase in drug therapy over recent years has resulted in medications being the most common cause of skin rashes. Drugs are ingested, injected, inhaled or even absorbed through the skin. The reactions are sudden, generalised, symmetrical and usually distant to the point of entry, as compared with the delayed localised reaction in contact dermatitis which is dealt with in the next chapter. The most frequent mechanism is a dermal vascular reaction resulting in erythema, with or without urticaria. There is usually also a fever within a few hours, often along with a generalised lymphadenopathy. A reaction may occur after many years of tolerance to the drug, and in a sensitised person it may even occur after intake of very small amounts.

The type of reaction to each drug may be either characteristic or non-specific. The characteristics include a generalised acute urticaria that can occur with penicillins, salicylates, quinine, and iodides which are contained in certain cough mixtures. Acute vesicular and bullous erythema may be caused by sulphonamides, phenobarbitone, iodides and bromides. Rashes resembling measles and scarlet fever can follow the use of barbiturates and also penicillins, sulphonamides and streptomycin. Some resembling lichen planus may be produced by gold, antimalarial (Fig. 30) and phenothiazine drugs, and those used for the treatment of cardiac arrhythmias and tuberculosis. Any drug can cause a rash that mimics polyarteritis nodosa or systemic lupus erythematosus, but this is rare.

Generalised exfoliative dermatitis is a potentially dangerous condition which can be caused by an allergy to sulphonamides, streptomycin or the heavy metals such as gold and arsenic. Light-sensitive eruptions occur at the areas exposed to the sun, often due to sensitivity to sulphonamides, tetracyclines, or the phenothiazine drugs.

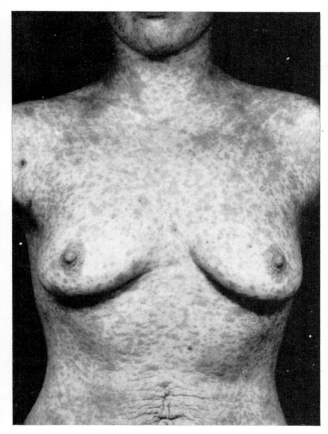

Fig. 30 Lichenoid drug eruption due to chloroquine.

Fixed drug eruptions can occur following the use of phenolphthalein which is contained in some laxatives but more rarely after barbiturates, salicylates, tartrazine food preservatives or sulphonamides. This reaction appears as a few localised patches, usually on the trunk or upper parts of the limbs. They are well circumscribed, lurid, dusky-red lesions, sometimes surmounted by a blister and usually lasting for a few days before leaving a hyperpigmented patch. The rash will usually reappear at the same site, following further ingestion of the drug.

A severe systemic upset can also follow drug sensitivity, the eruption being an exudative erythema multiforme (Stevens-Johnson syndrome). This may produce blisters and may even be fatal. Barbiturates can be the cause as well as long-acting tetracyclines and sulphonamides. These extensive problems need devoted nursing care and attention, as described towards the end of Chapter 9.

Pigmented purpuric dermatitis looks like a cross between dermatitis and purpura. The sedative carbromal is the usual cause but it is also seen with meprobamate. Cross-sensitivity between these two drugs has been reported.

Systemic penicillin is the commonest cause of a drug eruption, which can occur up to 4 weeks after cessation of treatment; like many others it can even pass to baby through mother's milk. Ampicillin commonly causes a rash when given to patients suffering from glandular fever. The antimalarial drug, chloroquine, occasionally causes bleaching of hair, as well as difficulty in focusing, photophobia and other eye symptoms; chloroquine retinopathy is irreversible. Sensitivity to barbiturates typically causes an erythematous or urticarial reaction, but also can produce purpuric, bullous or fixed eruptions as well as aphthus ulcers of the mouth and stomatitis. Chlorpromazine typically causes erythema, sometimes with a light sensitivity, and often with a cross-reaction with related drugs including other phenothiazine antihistamines and tranquillisers.

Bromides and iodides can cause an acneform rash which has no comedones. The chemicals are often contained in disinfectant lozenges, tonics and cough mixtures. Oral steroids can also cause an acneform eruption, as well as hirsutes and hyperpigmentation. Strong topical steroids can cause atrophy and degeneration of connective tissue, resulting in excessive bruising, as well as telangiectasia.

As drug reactions are potentially serious, an early diagnosis is made in the same way as in the urticarias, with close attention to details of dates and times. Identification is easier when the rash has a typical pattern caused by certain drugs. Some chemicals are more antigenic and therefore should always be thought of first.

A drug eruption should be suspected whenever there is an unidentified or unusual skin rash: for example, one looking like measles without Koplicks spots, conjunctivitis, or a premonitory upper respiratory infection. They should also be considered in all cases of exfoliative, vesicular or bullous lesions. On the legs, sulphonamides may produce symptoms similar to erythema nodosum.

Removal of the offending compound will result in a rapid drop in any pyrexia and in the disappearance of most rashes within a week; however, even a very minute amount of the chemical will cause relapse or prolongation of the lesions.

The taking of fluids should be encouraged to help removal of the drug by excretion. Tepid baths or sponging, but better still liberal applications of steroid creams, will bring symptomatic relief. Large doses of antihistamines will reduce further histamine release, allay symptoms and help prevent worsening of the rash due to scratching. Severe reactions may require systemic steroids and a careful watch on blood pressure and urine output; renal failure can occur. Subcutaneous adrenaline may be necessary.

Any known allergy should be recorded, and the drug and any closely related compounds should be strictly avoided. It is best that the patient understands this and knows to communicate the fact before being given any treatment; it is also a good idea for him to carry a card listing the compounds in case he is ever found in an unconscious state:

He was a well-known dentist who had first attended the clinic when he was 31 with a contact dermatitis of the fingers from an allergy to procaine. Changing the anaesthetic to lignocaine soon cleared the condition. It was surprising to see him 5 years later with contact dermatitis on his face. 'Oh, it's an actinic barrier lotion I was given; the rash came up after the first application.' The lotion contained para-aminobenzoic acid, which has the same antigenic para-amino grouping as the procaine to which he was already sensitised. 'Are there any other drugs to avoid?' 'Yes, you will probably be cross-sensitive to sulphonamides. There are now some chemotherapeutic combinations containing sulphonamide, such as co-trimoxazole. Sulphonamide rashes can be very severe, so do be careful.'

Chapter 8. Dermatitis

Any inflammation of the skin is called *dermatitis*. For simplicity in this book the term is used for rashes produced by external (exogenous) factors, while the term *eczema* is used when the causes are endogenous, as already described in Chapter 4. The histological changes in both conditions are identical. The problem is purely one of nomenclature but unfortunately there is no international agreement; some English dermatologists describe dermatitis under the term exogenous eczema. Dermatitis is important. It accounts for more than half the total time lost from industrial disease.

Dermatitis is due to contact with external physical agents and should be suspected in all cases involving a rash with an asymmetrical distribution, or when there is an acute exacerbation of an existing skin rash; the diagnosis is made from the history, distribution, pattern and shape (Fig. 31).

The condition is not infectious and this point should be emphasised to all sufferers; otherwise there is a tendency towards a preoccupation with dirt and germs, often resulting in the use of strong antiseptics which are guaranteed to worsen the condition. There are two main varieties: in allergic contact dermatitis, weak concentrations of antigenic substances produce a sensitivity reaction in the patient; in the other variety strong, abrasive, or repeatedly applied substances damage the skin. This type will be described first.

Primary irritant or traumatic dermatitis

The primary irritant or traumatic variety involves direct physical damage to the skin by mechanical or chemical factors. Most cases of dermatitis fall into this category.

Although each individual has a different susceptibility, irritants will cause inflammation in everyone, providing they are frequently applied and for long enough. Common culprits include acids, alkalis, antiseptics, abrasive dusts (such as stone, brick or coal), ultraviolet light,

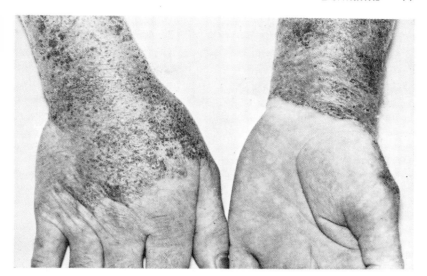

Fig. 31 Chronic dermatitis showing well-demarcated areas.

and extreme heat or cold. It is a matter of degree in that for example weak alkalis will cause a primary irritant dermatitis, whereas strong alkalis will result in the irreversible changes of a burn. 'Chapping' of exposed areas in cold weather is a traumatic dermatitis which occurs more readily in patients with a genetic tendency to ichthyosis (dry skin).

The skin is normally protected by a layer of sebum and the horny layer of keratin, which make it resistant to water and mild chemicals. Repeated washing with soap or detergents, however, causes degreasing with dryness, itching and then fissuring, with reduction of the skin's defences. Handling petrol (gasoline) and other fuels or solvents can have the same effect, as can the reduced sebum production in the aged. The hands are susceptible areas as they are frequently used and washed. This may be responsible for the development of the so-called 'house-wife's dermatitis'. The onset of the condition often follows childbirth because of the extra washing.

The ultraviolet portion of the light wavelengths is the most damaging to skin. It is filtered out by the atmosphere, dust, smoke and glass. Fair-skinned people are most susceptible to sunburn. Repeated exposure causes protective pigmentation and thickening of the skin. Further chronic exposure may lead to collagen degeneration (wrinkles), telangiectasia, and solar keratosis which may even progress to epithelioma. Unless protected by pigmented skin, years spent in the tropics inevitably take their toll. Ultraviolet light can also worsen psoriasis, lichen

planus, atopic eczema, and activate the virus herpes simplex (cold sores).
Light can also activate chemicals such as tar to cause contact dermatitis. The exposed areas are affected, such as the face, neck (but not under the chin), the 'V' area on the front of the chest, and the limbs. The condition is worse in the period between March and September in the northern hemisphere.

Allergic contact dermatitis

Allergic contact dermatitis is much more dramatic in its presentation. Minute quantities of the allergen will cause the reaction:

> He had been born in Iceland and had spent most of his 54 years fishing in the North Sea, where Dogger Bank Itch is well recognised amongst sailors. It is due to an allergy to the 'sea chervil' and occurs upon contact with the seaweed that is caught up in the nets. The dermatitis quickly clears on shore, but each successive attack is worse. There is weeping and swelling of the exposed areas of the hands and forearms and puffiness of the skin round the eyes; he tells a tale of having to prop his eyes open with matchsticks in order to see the compass! A very small patch test to the weed 3 years after stopping work was very strongly positive, and all the previously affected areas relapsed at the same time due to absorption. The true degree of his sensitivity was also shown by his story of waking up one night in his captain's cabin with irritation and swelling of the skin round the eyes, from the minute amount of the allergen in the air; on looking at his chart he found that he had been crossing the North Dogger.

Contact with the offending substance results in erythema, oedema and often an exudate; vesicles may appear and coalesce into bullae. The sensitivity is an acquired condition, which is rare before puberty and tends to appear or worsen during periods of physical or psychological illness. Sufferers may show cross-sensitivity to related compounds, in the same way as with allergy to drugs. The sensitivity usually lasts a lifetime, though it may diminish over the years. The effect upon the sufferer can be profound:

> The house was at the end of one of the valleys in the Lake District. It had been built long before dampcourses had been invented. The old lady brewed a lovely cup of tea, and always insisted that the postman came in and shared one with her. He hadn't the heart to tell her that each time by night fall he felt shivery, his skin started to irritate, and he knew he was in for an attack of his mould dermatitis. The consultant asked, 'Would you mind missing this lovely land of "mist and mellow fruitfulness" if you asked for a change to the sorting office where you

would not have this problem?' 'It would be worth it to lose my rash' was the reply.

Sensitivity can develop after many years of handling a substance without any previous ill-effect. It is a cell-mediated response, as described at the beginning of the next chapter, in which the antigen sensitises the 'T' lymphocytes (type IV hypersensitivity). The entire skin becomes sensitised and then a localised rash will occur at the sites of further contact. Either the offending substances are allergic in themselves, or are non-protein substances (Haptens) which combine with a skin protein to become an allergen.

Causes

The agents causing sensitisation include any substance under the sun (and including the sun!). In clothing, nickel is probably the worst culprit and is present in suspenders, buttons, zips, buckles and watch straps. Chemical dyes in materials are also common offenders, especially those used to colour nylon. Dermatitis can be caused by allergy to the rubber or elastic in gloves and hair nets, or to the rubber, leather, dyes or adhesives in shoes. Allergy can develop in those involved in manufacturing these compounds.

Cosmetics are a common cause of allergic contact dermatitis. These include hair dyes, lipstick, mascara, perfumes, hair lacquers and lanoline bases. Many household substances including detergents and polishes are potential allergens as they can easily penetrate the skin and cause sensitisation. Paint constituents such as resins and dyes, and chrome in the leather industry or as an impurity in cement can all cause the dermatitis, as may varnishes, adhesives and the additives in cutting or lubricating oils.

Medicaments applied locally can cause dermatitis. An existing eczema can be worsened by the development of sensitivity to topical applications. Common offenders include penicillin, neomycin, streptomycin, chlorpromazine, antihistamines, local anaesthetics especially procaine, and elastic adhesive plaster. Sensitised individuals may be unable to enter a room in which a drug is being handled without intense itching, swelling and scaling of the skin, especially around the eyes:

The 'phone rang after bedtime, which is unusual in a dermatologist's household! 'I'm going blind, the skin around my eyes is all swollen; what can I do?' It was the voice of the 30-year-old sister-in-charge on one of the wards for the mentally subnormal. Her patients were never good at taking tablets, so she crushed them up and had become sensitised 2 years previously. 'Have you had to handle chlorpromazine again?' 'Well, there was no-one else on duty, so I put on rubber gloves and gave the medicines out on a spoon.' 'What went wrong then?' 'A patient spat a tablet back into my face.'

Streptomycin can also have this effect in the form of droplets when the air from the syringe is sprayed into the atmosphere instead of into sterile cottonwool. Nurses must be taught to handle sensitisers with a strict no-touch technique. The chemicals are 'prickly' and must be avoided by the use of rubber gloves when repeated contact is necessary, otherwise the areas should be carefully washed with soap and water immediately after contact. Detergents and cleansers cause dryness of the skin, as has already been mentioned. This irritated skin is more easily damaged or sensitised to the compounds encountered in the nurse's duties. Streptomycin and antiseptics such as glutaraldehyde are

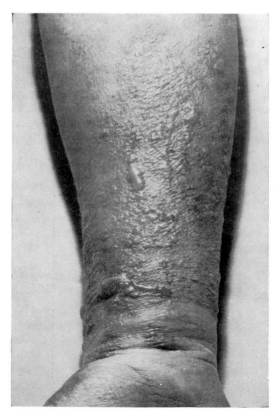

Fig. 32 Primula dermatitis showing vesicles in streaks from contact with the leaves.

particularly antigenic, and especially chlorpromazine in the presence of sunshine. If a nurse becomes sensitised to penicillin it means that she is denied the benefit of the many penicillin-based antibiotics for treatment of would-be fatal systemic infections.

Plants may cause allergic contact dermatitis. The most common one in England is the indoor primula obconica (Plate 17, Figs. 32, 33). (The outdoor primulas have no cross-sensitivity with the indoor variety.) In America the main problem is poison ivy. At the point of contact there is a violent vesicular reaction, often with a secondary urticaria of the face and neck. Other sensitisers include chrysanthemums, tulips, daffodils, narcissi and celery. Hogweed, cow parsley, herbs such as dill, as well as vegetables (celery and parsnips) can cause a light-sensitive (phytophoto) dermatitis. These plants come from the same family (*Umbilleferae*) from which psoralen is obtained for the treatment of psoriasis by PUVA as described on page 192. It is of interest that a compound causing a local sensitivity reaction can also produce iatrogenic disease internally; chloramphenicol may cause contact dermatitis when used locally or agranulocytosis when given systemically. But it may be life saving in haemophilus influenzae meningitis or typhoid fever.

Affected areas

The areas affected in dermatitis are initially those of contact with the

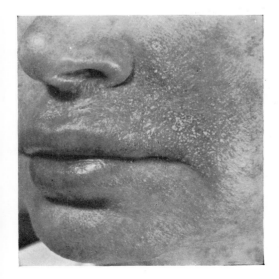

Fig. 33 Primula dermatitis, the allergen being spread to the face by nose picking. (Same patient as Fig. 32.)

offending substance. Swelling and scaling of the eyelids and surrounding skin should be considered to be due to contact dermatitis until proved otherwise (Fig. 34). This is because this site is very susceptible to airborne allergens including pollens, moulds and dusts. Small quantities may also be carried to the site when patients rub their eyes; nail varnish is an example. The ears can react to topical antibiotics or to the plastic or metal of spectacles. Cosmetics and soaps will affect their points of contact. The scalp may become allergic to any local application, and spread may then take place to the ears, face and even shoulders. Allergy to hair dye would affect the same areas:

> The rash certainly had an odd distribution—just on the left upper anterior surface of his chest. It varied considerably, being much worse when he was working 'long hours', and clearing up on the family holidays. He was 43. However, the story went deeper than the apparent stress connection; a patch test showed him to be sensitive to a particular hair dye, whereas his firm handled only grain. He was asked if his wife dyed her hair; the consultation was terminated by an abrupt 'certainly not!'. The young registrar was puzzled, so he telephoned the patient's family doctor. There was a long chuckle at the other end of the line; 'Yes, most of his firm live here in the village and are my patients, so are well known to me. I can tell you the colour of the hair dye to which he is sensitive!'

The axilla is susceptible to dermatitis from deodorants and antiperspirants. The hands are often affected, commonly by soaps, detergents, petrols, oils, and irritants such as cement. Irritants and sensi-

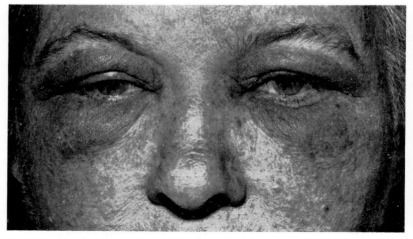

Fig. 34   Allergic contact dermatitis showing swelling and scaling.

tisers affect the areas where the skin is thinnest, such as the clefts and backs of the fingers and hands. The palms are usually spared as the skin is thicker. Substances become concentrated under rings and are less easily washed away; allergy to the nickel in cheap or soldered gold is not uncommon.

The trunk may also be affected by clothing, especially of the drip-dry variety. Allergy to contraceptives can directly affect the genitals. Rashes on legs are typically caused by elastic, elasticated nylon, or the dyes of stockings or socks (Figs. 35, 36). As already mentioned, shoes

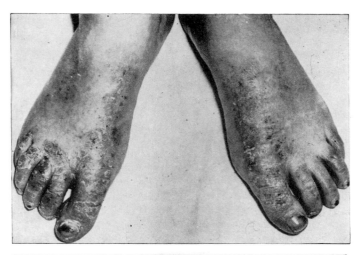

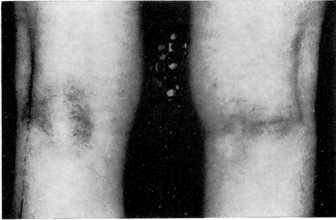

Figs. 35 & 36 Dermatitis from nylon tights showing the two main sites affected.

can cause a dermatitis of the feet; this has to be distinguished from tinea infections, as discussed from page 121. Eruptions mainly affecting the insteps are more likely to be caused by endogenous rather than exogenous factors, but patch tests must always be carried out when the dorsa (backs) of the feet are involved.

It should be pointed out that dermatitis of the hands can be due to secondary absorption from nickel dermatitis elsewhere, as already discussed on page 43. The original site may have cleared, leaving the hands still affected. Any patients suffering from incurable hand dermatitis should always be given nickel sulphate 25 mg by mouth, as a flare-up of the rash would be suggestive of allergy.

Allergen identification

Identification of the allergen requires the taking of an accurate history. This should include the patient's occupation and hobbies, and whether others doing the same job are similarly affected. Variations of the dermatitis should be noted, such as the rapid improvement after a weekend away from work or a holiday away from home. An accurate diary record of what the patient does and how the skin varies is probably the best single method of investigating sensitivity rashes. The incubation time between contact and exacerbation of the rash is within a day. Careful perusal of the diary usually gives the answer. If not, then seeing the patient in his own surroundings, whether at work or at home, may be necessary to ascertain detailed information that even the most diligent historian might miss.

In conjunction with the history, however, the location of the rash may make the identification much easier. For example, the apex of the axilla is usually involved in allergies to antiperspirants and deodorants, but is normally spared in sensitivity to clothing.

As in all dermatology conditions, clinical inspection should always include normal as well as abnormal skin. Full examination of the undressed patient is usually needed to see the rash in its entirety:

> It was the aerial movement of a flock of wader birds that was so fascinating to watch—twisting and turning, then spreading out to skim over the bay. The young landlady approached and said, 'Are you watching the winter migration, doctor? I've a rash all round my trunk, it has just come out. Can you give me anything?' 'Well you can't strip off here,' observed the consultant! Examination was suggested in more professional surroundings. The rash was erythematous and scaling. It was well demarcated in a band round the breasts and back. The areas corresponded exactly to certain parts of her bra' where it contained an elastic material. It would not have been possible, without full examination, to diagnose that she was allergic to elasticated nylon.

Patch testing should only be undertaken when the skin is in a quiescent phase. 'AL' test rolls or Finn chambers on microporous adhesive tape can be used. A very small amount of the substance to be tested is applied to a white absorbent disc or into a Finn chamber and placed upon an area of normal skin, usually on the patient's back. The aluminium backing provides occlusion, and is held in place by adhesive tape. A standard battery of the common allergens is now commercially available (Fig. 37). Each test should be identified by marking the patient's skin; a fine cottonwool applicator dipped in dihydroxyacetone 5% or crystal violet 0.5% in spirit, or alternatively a crystal violet pencil should be used for this purpose.

Patients must be told to remove the strips and wash the area only if there is pain or undue irritation. Otherwise the tests must be left alone and water avoided. The strips are usually removed by the nurse or doctor at 48 hours. The patient must then wait half an hour before the tests are read. Erythema at the site denotes possible sensitivity, whereas a spreading erythema or a patch of dermatitis is conclusive. The tests should also be read 2 days later, as a delayed positive result may then have appeared; erythema or dermatitis persisting at this time is again diagnostic of a sensitivity. Reference books such as *Contact Dermatitis* by Fisher, or *Textbook of Dermatology* by Rook, Wilkinson and

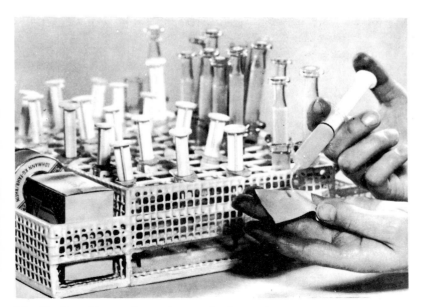

Fig. 37 Portable tray for storing standard test substances.

Ebling (3rd edition, 1979; Blackwell Scientific Publications, Oxford), should be consulted for further details of patch-test readings. The strength of any other substance to be investigated can be obtained from comprehensive lists in the reference books just mentioned. Applying the substance in too strong a concentration causes a primary irritant reaction and therefore a false positive result. If the concentration is too weak, a false negative result may occur, as can also happen when a case of photosensitivity dermatitis is investigated without ultraviolet light.

Management

The management of contact dermatitis involves re-educating the patient to avoid the offending substance, in all its forms and disguises. The word 'patient' describes a transitory phase in a person's life, and it is well to remember that most nurses and doctors at some time become patients as well! If admitted patients must be encouraged to take an active part in the ward routines, in order to prevent deterioration of morale. The word 'dermatitis' is dreaded by lay people because it is believed to be a chronic condition which will prevent them from ever being able to work again. If you discuss the diagnosis with them it is wise to use the term 'exogenous eczema'. However, there are some patients who will welcome the chance to claim compensation and this also encourages chronicity.

Patients must avoid all contact with the offending substance. Unfortunately this is usually for life, although in time a reduction of sensitivity may take place. General advice to the patient should include not handling degreasing agents, using soap sparingly, and regularly applying emollients after washing. Barrier creams should be used when possible; they only slightly reduce contact with sensitisers, but do make it easier to remove irritants and dirty oils from the skin after work. In this regard industrial skin cleansers such as Swarfega are also helpful.

Contact with irritants can be avoided by the use of aprons, boots and gloves. The use of long-handled mops and other kitchen aids, such as dish and clothes washers should be encouraged. Patients who are sensitive to elastic adhesive plaster, can dress any injury with microporous tape, tubular dressings or even an acrylic resin spray.

New workers can develop transient rashes as their skin becomes accustomed to meeting new substances; the process is known as 'hardening'. Adequate dust extraction and ventilation will prevent the accumulation of irritants. A happy worker in good working conditions is less likely to develop contact dermatitis. Adequate protection against the traumatic forms of dermatitis may enable a sufferer to return to the same job, but this is not usually possible when there is contact sensitivity.

It is better to clear the patient's skin by removing him from the source of his problem but at the same time keeping him at work. This method is good for morale and discourages 'compensationitis'. Chronicity can only be prevented if the skin is completely cleared. A workman with residual scaling of his finger clefts from an attack 5 years previously will have the same tendency to chronicity as if he had had dermatitis for the whole period. It is mandatory that the skin texture and patterning of all affected areas become normal before therapy is stopped.

Treatment

Acute contact dermatitis can often be cleared by simply removing the offending agent. Further treatment is aimed at reducing the inflammation, but without adding any possible irritants or sensitisers. Desensitisation courses have not been found to be successful.

The first line of treatment is the use of bland preparations, such as wet dressings of inert lotions which cool by evaporation, the remaining inert powder absorbing any exudate. These are very useful, especially for large areas, and include calamine lotion BP. Daily cleaning with cooking oil is usually required to soften and remove any dried lotion.

Steroid preparations are the mainstay of treatment. In the acute stages they should be applied 3 or 4 times a day, reducing to daily; a weaker preparation should then be used for at least 2 weeks after complete clearance of the rash. This lessens the chance of a recurrence once treatment has ceased. The use of a bland tar ointment for a few weeks after return to work is also helpful and protective; calamine and coal tar ointment BPC is a suitable preparation.

Dressings should separate all skin surfaces to prevent any painful adherence, and should be changed before they dry out. Oedema worsens any weeping, and can be reduced by bed rest and elevation of the affected part; dry gauze dressings are then all that are needed. Tense blisters should be opened with sterile scissors but the roof allowed to remain as a natural dressing.

Painful cracks will develop if the lesions become overdried. This can be prevented by the application of zinc and salicylic acid paste BP (Lassar's Paste) covered with tubular gauze, or old nylon stockings or tights. In cold weather the paste should be softened before application by placing the container in a warm place. When there is secondary infection, potassium permanganate 1 : 8000 baths or soaks give good symptomatic relief. Systemic antibiotics are sometimes needed. In severe cases, wearing cotton gloves day and night is also useful as a conscious reminder to the patient to avoid any contact. When the hands are in water, these gloves should be covered with loose-fitting plastic overgloves.

Lichenified dermatitis should first be treated with topical steroids. These should be used as in the treatment of eczema, described on page 46. Prolonged use causes side-effects, as detailed on page 211, and therefore resistant cases require impregnated bandages, usually coal tar paste or zinc paste BP—these can be left in place covered with tubular gauze or elastic adhesive plaster for 1–2 weeks. Impregnated bandages used in this manner have the added psychological advantage of hiding the lesions.

Repeated attacks of dermatitis are not only demoralising for the patient but actually weaken the skin's resistance against the normal irritants encountered in everyday life. The patient should therefore always be cleared as quickly as possible and education given to prevent relapse.

When light causes the dermatitis, it must be completely avoided until the rash is cleared. This includes reflected as well as direct light and also that from fluorescent tubes. When clear, patients can be allowed to go outside provided that they are adequately protected; clothing should cover as much of the body as possible and, for example, sandals should not be worn without socks. Wide-brimmed hats are mandatory but unpopular. Yellow soft paraffin, red veterinary petroleum jelly (red vet. pet.) or inert substances such as titanium dioxide will absorb or deflect light. Certain specialised formulations absorb specific wavelengths. Creams are available containing mexenone (Uvistat) or its derivatives (Delial 10) and also a lotion containing padimate (Spectroban).

Antimalarial drugs have a limited part to play in the more severe conditions. Oral Mepacrine is probably the safest, but patients have to put up with the fact that it turns the skin a dirty yellow.

Patients with chronic dermatitis may become light-sensitive and this aggravates and perpetuates the eruption; the condition is called actinic reticuloid. The whole skin may then become involved as a generalised exfoliative dermatitis; this is important from the nursing point of view, as the patient must be admitted to hospital. As the condition is light-sensitive the patients have to be nursed in a darkened room, lit only by an ordinary light bulb.

Other causes of generalised exfoliative dermatitis include drugs such as sulphonamides, malignancy especially the reticuloses, and pre-existing eczema or lichen planus often after a treatment reaction (exfoliative psoriasis has already been considered on page 15). The whole skin is dusky red, irritable and scaling; lymphadenopathy and oedema occur throughout the body. Secondary infection causes crusting. The increased blood flow may result in heart failure in the elderly, requiring appropriate treatment. Hair and nail loss is common. Treatment in a controlled temperature is necessary, with the use of a low-reading thermometer to monitor heat loss. A high-protein diet should be given, and a close watch must be made for malnutrition as the gut lining may also be affected.

Treatment of the underlying cause is necessary. Oral steroids, such as prednisolone in a reducing daily dose from 60 mg, are effective to-gether with local steroids applied by the handful! Quicker results follow combined internal and external therapy as is so often the case in dermatology. Secondary sepsis is controlled by giving antibiotics systemically or adding econazole 0.25 % to the steroid ointment.

The presence of an extensive rash causes much anxiety with con-sequent worsening of the eruption; full nursing therapy along with reassurance that the condition can be cleared are both essential to reverse the process:

He looked much older than 55, and had retired early because of his skin complaint. He had started work as a lad in the iron ore smelter, but had changed to heavy engineering when the foundry was closed. Although a reliable worker, he found the change to the lathe with its grease quite difficult at the age of 51. Two years later his hands started to chap, for which he blamed the severe winter. The weather improved but the chapping worsened. Small red areas appeared between the fingers and in the clefts, and spread over the backs of the hands with weeping, crusting and irritation. He did his best to continue, but the foreman sent him to his doctor. He was given a medical certificate. On it was the word 'dermatitis'. 'You felt as if you had been kicked by a horse. All your life's work come to nothing; you were ready for the knacker's yard!' After a fortnight at home, the rash was greatly improved but not cleared so he stopped treatment and was foolishly allowed to start work again. All went well for a month, but relapse slowly occurred. It was better after a weekend at home or a short holiday. It improved when he used treatment at work, but he couldn't get enough ointment to put on after washing his hands. The periods of sickness became longer, the rash worsening more quickly and spreading more extensively each time he returned to work. Sensitivity to daylight then developed, and ultimately all areas of his skin were covered with a weeping, generalised exfoliative dermatitis. He was hypothermic.
'Can you do anything for me at all?'
Events had nearly broken him, but there was dignity in his gaze. He was

told that admission into a darkened but really warm room in hospital would be arranged. If he wanted the condition to clear more quickly, he would have to be treated with some messy crystal violet and steroid ointment to stop him from rubbing and worsening his skin. By now he was shivering but looked reassured.

'You can use whatever colour you like, but what about the nurses' hands and the sheets?' he asked. 'The sheets are no problem as we use disposable or green ones. Because of the effectiveness of the treatment the nurses don't mind using it; it will be the only time you will see them wearing gloves. In 2 months' time you will be clear.'

Chapter 9. Immunology, blistering diseases

The body controls its growth and replacement by a remarkable number of interrelated mechanisms. This must include the ability to recognise its own cells but destroy and engulf foreign substances and infective agents. The same mechanisms may be involved in the control of cancer. The majority of the blistering diseases that have systemic origins are due to immunological processes, and are dealt with later in this chapter from dermatitis herpetiformis onwards.

Immunology

Immunology involves both an antibody and a cellular response to invasion. An allergy is an excessive response to these circumstances. In the autoimmune diseases the body fails to 'recognise' its own tissues and makes antibodies against them, with ultimate damage to the organ or organs in question. The immune response has been touched upon briefly in previous chapters but, for those readers who are interested, the subject is covered here in a little more depth.

The cells involved with immunity are a type of white cell called lymphocytes. These include the humoral type known as B cells, which produce and release antibodies called immunoglobulins. This is in response to a specific foreign substance called an antigen. On becoming attached to this antigen, the antibodies will bring about either disintegration, neutralisation of any toxicity, or enhanced identification and engulfing of the antigen by macrophage cells.

The other main group of lymphocytes are involved in the cell-mediated type of immunity and are called T cells. These are best described as 'killer cells', acting against other cells which may be either foreign to the body as in the case of organ transplants or against body cells which have been altered; this can be caused by viruses such as measles or mumps, or by chemicals including the antigens of contact dermatitis.

There are various other lymphocytes, including those concerned with immunological memory which are responsible for the persistence and control.

Allergens vary from medicines, chemicals, metals, proteins and bacterial toxins, to bacteria and pollens. Sensitisation, which is the building up or initiation of an immunity, occurs after a minimum of about 4 days and usually lasts indefinitely. When the allergen is a dead or attenuated bacteria or virus, as in inoculations, the procedure is known as *active* immunisation. When an antiserum is used, which is a specimen of sensitised blood from another individual or animal who has been previously exposed to the antigen, it is known as *passive* immunisation.

Patients with allergies usually have a positive family history, often showing atopy, as discussed previously. They may also show an abnormally high level of a particular antibody called IgE (reaginic antibody). The release of histamine and related compounds is due to the combination of the antigen and this antibody, and systemically may result in a severe and occasionally fatal reaction. There are often associated pyrexia, sweating, malaise, diarrhoea and vomiting.

If the allergen reaction is localised and at the area of contact between the antibody and antigen, the site is called a shock organ. If this is the skin then pruritus or the urticarias will occur, whereas if it is the nasal mucosa or the bronchioles then there is hay-fever or asthma respectively. If the blood vessels are involved then an arteritis is produced as in erythema multiforme.

There are four types of excessive immune response which do occur and can be harmful; the first three of these hypersensitivity reactions are antibody mediated, immediate types, whereas the fourth is a cell-mediated, delayed reaction.

Type 1

Type 1 (anaphylaxis) occurs when the IgE antibody and antigen complex causes a release of histamine and related substances. If the shock organ is localised then for example urticaria, asthma or hay-fever will occur. If the reaction is generalised, as following an injection or a bite, then laryngeal oedema and skin rashes may occur, along with the bronchospasm; there may be a sudden fall in blood pressure and even death.

Desensitisation may be effective against systemic but not localised type 1 reactions; frequent injections of very small amounts of the antigen will cause a rise in an appropriate antibody of a different type, namely IgG. This is not fixed in the tissues as IgE, and can therefore mop up the antigen before it reaches the latter.

Type 2

Type 2 reactions are antibody-mediated cytolytic or cytotoxic types, as an incompatible blood transfusions, haemolytic disease of the newborn (Rhesus incompatibility), and the autoimmune haemolytic anaemias.

Type 3

Type 3 reactions can be local or systemic. The Arthus reaction occurs at the site of contact in a previously sensitised individual where there is a local excess of antigen, resulting in oedema and petechial haemorrhage. Conversely, serum sickness occurs when there is an excess of antibody, for example when the antitetanus horse serum passive inoculation is being slowly released into the blood of a previously sensitised individual. This systemic reaction can be dangerous when it involves the heart and kidneys. When present in equal concentrations antigen-antibody complexes can cause microprecipitates around small blood vessels, which produce inflammation and their blockage, as in post streptococcal anaphylactoid purpura (Henoch Schoenlein) or glomerular nephritis.

Type 4

Type 4 is the T cell-mediated, delayed reaction which becomes apparent from 12 to 48 hours after a second contact with the antigen. In it there is a migration of lymphocytes and macrophages into the tissues, hence the delay. The antigens are either foreign cells, such as in the rejection of a transplanted organ or skin grafts, or ordinary cells which have been altered; this modification occurs when certain materials combine with cell-wall proteins and become antigenically active as substances called haptens. This can occur following the topical application of antibiotics, or contact with primulas, nickel or chrome, as described in Chapter 8 as the allergic form of dermatitis.

Blisters

Blisters are very upsetting for the patient because of their appearance and soreness. In the days of the Old Testament Job's problems lasted 7 years, but the prognosis has improved since those days! The nurse can do much to comfort and reassure if she knows something about their natural history and treatment of the disorders that cause them. Blisters due to drugs have already been mentioned, but reference books should be consulted for an exhaustive classification of all causes.

Impetigo is usually due to a staphylococcus, and like other skin infections can blister; this especially occurs in the newborn, in debilitated children, in the tropics, and when the condition is inadvertently treated with local steroids. Impetigo is discussed in greater detail on page 115. Herpes simplex and zoster also cause vesicles (small blisters).

Burns, scalds and frostbite

Burns, scalds and frostbite can cause extensive blistering, depending on the degree of damage. Even sunburn can blister. Their local treatments are similar and are described on page 211.

Dermatitis herpetiformis

Dermatitis herpetiformis is a rare but very irritable eruption. The blisters are small and occur on the forearms, thighs, upper back, lumbosacral regions and round the scalp. There are associated erythematous areas (Fig. 38) and pigmentation from previous lesions. There is usually an associated glutenenteropathy, with flattening of the jejunal mucosa as in coeliac disease. The last-mentioned disorder is due to an allergy to gluten proteins which are present in wheat and other grains. 'Contact dermatitis of the small gut' is an oversimplification; however,

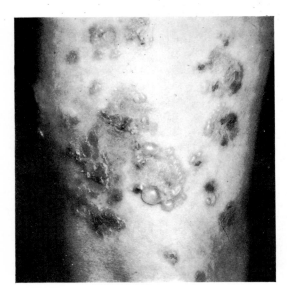

Fig. 38 Dermatitis herpetiformis showing small tense blisters arising from erythematous areas.

it does emphasise how interrelated all the parts of the body are and that no single organ can be completely considered in isolation.

A gluten-free diet is helpful in most cases of dermatitis herpetiformis, but as it is bland many patients prefer treatment with dapsone. This drug is so effective that it can be used as a therapeutic test. Dapsone occasionally causes anaemia and the patients may look cyanosed due to methaemoglobinaemia and sulphaemoglobinaemia. Sulphapyridine may then have to be used as an alternative drug. After satisfactory control for a few months the dosage can be slowly reduced and then varied as required.

Pemphigoid

Pemphigoid, like dermatitis herpetiformis, presents with tense blisters but they are larger and occur in an older age group. The shins may be affected first, and later the arms and trunk; the blisters often contain blood and arise from irritable ring-shaped erythematous areas (Fig. 39). Admission to hospital is necessary to initiate treatment with

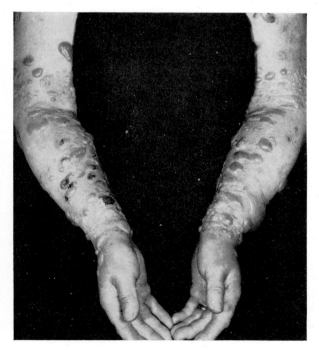

Fig. 39 Pemphigoid showing characteristic tense blisters.

prednisolone and an antimitotic drug such as azathiaprine. Some cases may be due to internal malignancy; all patients should be carefully examined clinically, blood tests performed including the ESR or plasma viscosity, and five consecutive stools examined for the presence of occult blood. It is a question of clinical judgement as to how much a frail old person should be subjected to further examinations; 'Thou shalt not kill nor strive officiously to keep alive' is an old adage to be remembered. On the other hand, carcinoma discovered radiologically by barium enema in these patients has a better prognosis than for other sites.

Dermatological nursing for this condition can be as life-saving as in pemphigus, which is described in greater detail on page 97. The large blisters should be drained but the roof left as a dressing. If the patient is fit enough, a saline with potassium permanganate bath may ease symptoms. Repeated reassurance and encouragement are required but above all patience is essential:

> He was brilliant in his research work but useless as head of a
> department. Promotion and administration unfortunately go hand in
> hand. He resented battling for research funds. At 40 years of age he was
> an international figure in his own right. Why did his firm not
> acknowledge this and give him the money to complete his work?
> Red areas erupted firstly on the shins but then on the limbs and finally
> the trunk, with many tense blisters some of which were haemorrhagic.
> Urgent admission was arranged. The patient was as upset about not
> doing his research as he was about the appalling state of his skin. His
> agitation was barely controlled by heavy sedation, and the soreness of
> the rash by phenoxyethanol 2% in hydrocortisone ointment.
> A clinical diagnosis of pemphigoid was made; after biopsy of an entire
> blister, and serology to detect antibasement membrane antibodies,
> prednisolone and azathioprine were given. Contrary to expectations, the
> condition was little changed a fortnight later. The dosage was increased
> and the advice of a world figure sought at a dermatology meeting; he
> confirmed that nothing more could be done. It was only after persisting
> with the treatment that the pemphigoid was brought under control, but
> by then the drugs had caused hypertension.

Pemphigus

In the pre-steroid era pemphigus carried more than a 90% mortality. Prednisolone in a daily dosage of up to 180 mg, together with an antimitotic drug, usually controls the condition, but not unexpectedly the treatment occasionally has fatal side-effects.

In pemphigus the blisters tend to start near to or in the mouth or the anogenital region but later spread extensively. The patients are younger than in pemphigoid (Fig. 40). The blisters are more superficial and

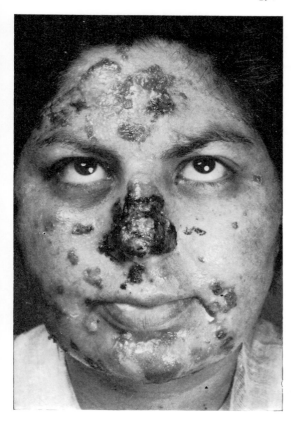

Fig. 40 Pemphigus showing characteristic superficial blisters near orifices.

flaccid (Plate 18). Histologically the split can be seen within the epidermis itself with the presence of acantholytic cells, whereas in pemphigoid and dermatitis herpetiformis the split is subepidermal. There are other differentiating features including the presence of antibodies in the patient's serum against the intercellular substance of epithelial cells in pemphigus; in pemphigoid antibodies against the basement membranes are usually found.

The patients are acutely uncomfortable and need twice-daily applications of soothing mildly antiseptic steroid ointment in large quantities; the one favoured is phenoxyethanol 2% in hydrocortisone ointment. Cross-infection must be prevented by barrier nursing. The skin is sometimes so sore that it is kinder to put the ointment lavishly on strips of soft old cotton sheet and use these as dressings directly on the skin; alternatively absorbent nonadherent foam dressings covered with tubular cotton gauze can be used. Dressings should be repeated whenever the areas become sore and dry. Analgesics should be given an hour before each dressing.

Oral hygiene is important. Soluble salicylate gels such as Bonjela seem to give the most symptomatic relief, sometimes in conjunction with crystal violet 0.5% in water, depending on the organisms cultured; amphotericin B lozenges or nystatin pessaries slowly sucked may be needed to control the overgrowth of yeasts from oral steroids, immunosuppressants and antibiotics.

The nursing of pemphigus is a great challenge. The patients are sore and ill; they are obviously distressed about their plight and need comfort and reassurance. Detailed attention to all the physical treatments, together with a compassionate approach, is essential.

Erythema multiforme

Erythema multiforme is drug induced in about one-third of all cases, and viral in origin in the rest. The characteristic lesion is the 'shooting target' (Fig. 41) with a dark centre and surrounding differing shades of red. 'Toxic' sites are affected, such as the extremities, where the circulation is slower. In the exudative or severe form (Stevens-Johnson syndrome) the centres of the lesions blister and coalesce. Most of the limbs and body are involved but also the mouth, lips, conjunctivae and much of the respiratory tract. It is sometimes necessary to give the

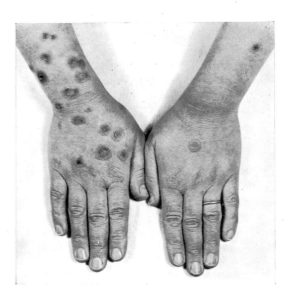

Fig. 41 Erythema multiforme showing characteristic target lesions.

massive dosage of steroids by injection if the patient cannot swallow. Real dermatological nursing, with emphasis on the patient's comfort and the avoidance of cross-infection, is mandatory:

He had suffered a severe coronary thrombosis only 3 months previously and the anticoagulant phenindione had been given. Urgent admission to hospital had to be arranged as most of his skin had suddenly developed circular red areas (Plate 19). He was sore, despondent and very ill. He looked much older than 49. The mouth was the worst area with so many sore erosions. Occasionally he coughed up large pieces that were obviously the lining of the trachea and larger bronchi. 'I think it's beating me, doctor.' The consultant tried to be reassuring, but was dispirited as he feared the steroids he was giving might precipitate another coronary. It was before the days of gentamicin. One wonders now if the drug would have prevented his ultimate and unpleasant death from pseudomonas bronchopneumonia. Severe Stevens-Johnson syndrome carries a high mortality.

Chapter 10. Cutaneous manifestations of systemic disease and malignancy

Systemic disease

Many medical conditions have skin manifestations: the bronzed colour of haemochromatosis, the dark skin of adrenal cortical insufficiency, the puce colour of polycythaemia, or the obvious yellow of jaundice. As would be expected more than one organ is often affected in systemic disease; it is therefore of great use to examine the skin carefully for diagnostic clues as to what is happening elsewhere.

The autoimmune diseases are the most colourful; most of them show evidence of 'C' shaped vascular patterning on the skin (livido reticularis) together with small arteritic ulcers, or telangiectasia at the bases of the nails. Vascular collagen is mainly involved and this is why previously they were known as the collagen diseases: lupus erythematosus, dermatomyositis, polyarteritis nodosa and rheumatoid disease. These conditions can be differentiated by clinical as well as chemical observations. Treatment is by large doses of systemic steroids and immunosuppressants; they are not considered further in this book as dermatological nursing is not usually an important facet of their treatment. In the really acute stages of the illness patients do of course need the same comfort, rest and support as mentioned in the previous chapter.

Chronic discoid lupus erythematosus

Chronic discoid lupus erythematosus is the quiescent autoimmune variety and rarely becomes acute and systemic. Characteristically it affects exposed surfaces such as the 'butterfly' areas of the face (cheeks and nose), and less often the scalp or mucosae (Plate 20). The affected areas are red and follicular, and if the adherent scale is removed characteristic 'tin tacks' of keratin can be seen projecting downwards. The lesions tend to extend at the margin and heal in the centre, leaving a slightly depressed scar; on the scalp they have an irregular surface whereas in lichen planus they are smooth. Both conditions cause a scarring alopecia which is permanent.

Treatment should be with a very strong topical steroid; it must be applied accurately to the lesion in order to prevent damage of the surrounding normal skin. The treatment can be intensified by applying plastic adhesive strapping over the ointment and this may be left in position for a few days at a time. The steroid flurandrenolone (Haelan) is available as a tape that can be cut to size.

Many of the patients' lesions are made worse by daylight. The plasters, the ointment base itself, or the cosmetic powders applied on top are all suitable actinic barriers. Mepacrine or chloroquine by mouth also reduce actinic sensitivity. These may be needed in some instances, but the former drug stains all the skin a dirty yellow and the latter may damage the eyes. Patients with eruptions that are worsened by actinic rays always seem to forget about their sensitivity. It is often necessary to give them written instructions to protect themselves from daylight by wearing a wide-brimmed hat, long sleeves, high necks and slacks.

Systemic sclerosis

Systemic sclerosis (systemic scleroderma) is a rare condition in which the changes of Raynaud's phenomenon progress to an atrophy, sclerosis and vasculitis of internal organs as well as of the skin (Figs. 42a, b). Ulceration and loss of the extremities occurs. The condition follows a progressive course invariably terminating in death, usually due to intercurrent infection, heart or renal failure. It is believed to be autoimmune in origin and mostly affects adult females. There is a characteristic progressive development of stiff, hard skin, making movement of small joints difficult, and producing a characteristic contracted expressionless visage, with a beaked nose and radial furrows round the mouth. Mastication and closing the hands eventually become impossible. Characteristic telangiectatic tufts are often present in the sclerotic areas which may calcify.

Localised scleroderma

Localised scleroderma (morphea) is not of systemic importance unless it strikes through to bone and causes hemiatrophy, which is fortunately very rare. Otherwise the thick areas of skin are only a cosmetic problem. Strong steroid ointments give relief if there is irritation.

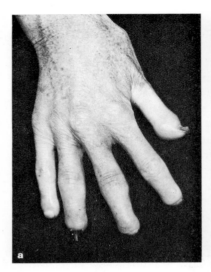 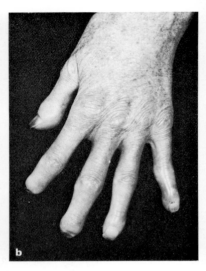

Fig. 42a & b   Systemic sclerosis showing tapered sclerotic fingers.

Lichen sclerosis et atrophicus

Lichen sclerosis et atrophicus is thought to be a superficial form of localised scleroderma. It is an important condition only when it affects the skin of the glans penis or labia (Fig. 43). Leukoplakia can then follow with the ultimate possibility of carcinoma (Fig. 44); regular biopsies are usually needed to exclude this development. Early and regular use of strong steroid preparations usually causes resolution of the 'scleroderma', leaving a pink atrophy from treatment. Careful follow up is still needed.

Xanthomata

Xanthomata are yellow, waxy nodular cholesterol deposits on the extensor surfaces and round the eyes. Their cosmetic treatment is mentioned on page 182 but it is more important to ascertain why they are present. They may be due to hyperlipidaemia or even diabetes, and both of these are associated with vascular disease which may ultimately prove fatal.

Pruritus

Pruritus (itching) may be due to anaemia, uraemia, endocrine conditions, liver disease including secondary deposits and overt malignancy;

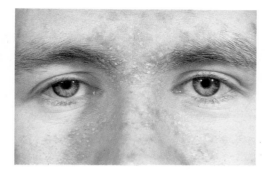

Plate 1 Psoriasis of face appearing 1 week after being jilted.

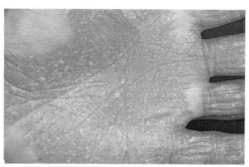

Plate 2 Psoriasis of palm developing in a man nursing his wife through her terminal illness; the soles and other palm were similarly affected.

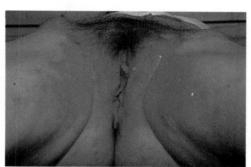

Plate 3 Flexural psoriasis showing localised scaling salmon-coloured eruption; the patient's history is given on page 67.

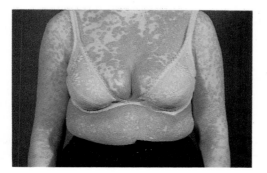

Plate 4 Widespread unstable psoriasis following the use of strong local steroids.

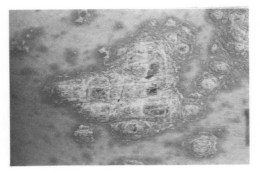

Plate 5 Psoriasis actively erupting and spreading; these early lesions are more pink than the quiescent one shown in Plate 6.

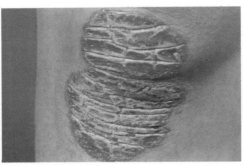

Plate 6 Psoriasis showing a characteristic salmon-coloured quiescent plaque covered with silvery scales that stop short of the edge.

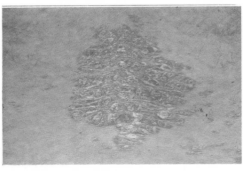

Plate 7 Psoriasis before treatment.

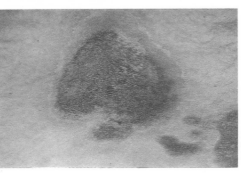

Plate 8 Reduction in the thickness of the lesion as the dithranol stain develops. Five applications of the stiff ointment have been made.

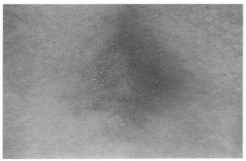

Plate 9 Psoriasis cleared after ten applications, the dithranol stain remaining.

Plate 10 Two weeks later when the stain has disappeared.

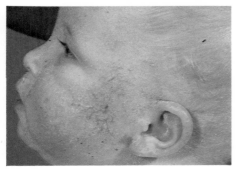

Plate 11 Infantile eczema showing typical excoriated scaling areas.

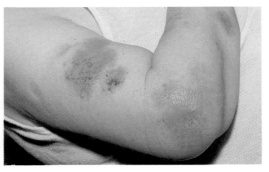

Plate 12 Discoid eczema with excoriations.

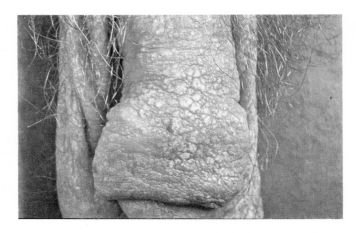

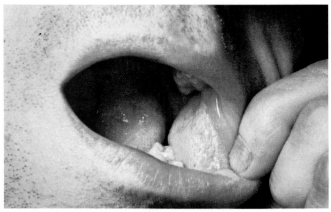

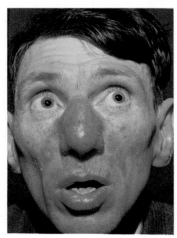

Plate 13 (*top*) Lichen planus showing typical lilac-coloured polygonal papules.

Plate 14 (*centre*) Lichen planus of inner cheek.

Plate 15 (*left*) Rosacea showing gross erythema with some pustules and papules. (Unrelated, note the patient's expression as he is also mentally subnormal.)

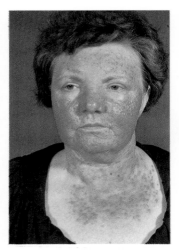

Plate 16 Rosacea made more extensive, papular and florid by the use of strong local steroids.

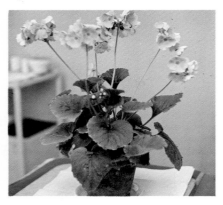

Plate 17 Primula obconica, the commonest cause of contact dermatitis from plants in Britain.

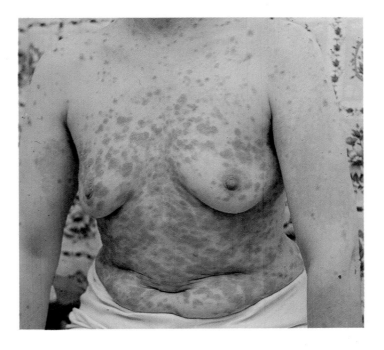

Plate 18 Pemphigus vulgaris in the early stages showing numerous superficial erosions.

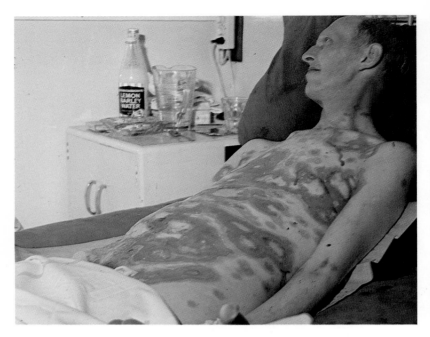

Plate 19 Extensive Stevens-Johnson syndrome showing extensive red areas and typical smaller 'target' lesions on the flanks; the patient's history is given on page 99.

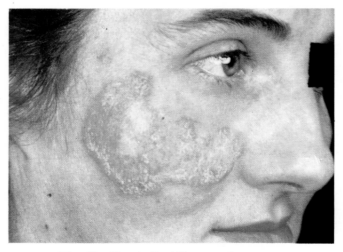

Plate 20 Chronic discoid lupus erythematosus.

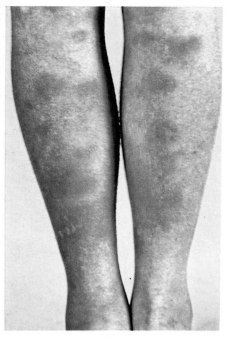

Plate 21 Erythema nodosum showing typical red tender raised areas, mainly circular.

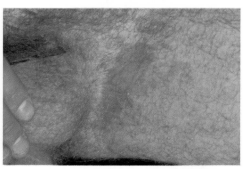

Plate 22 Erythrasma showing characteristic localised fine scaling areas.

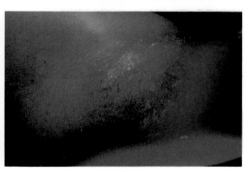

Plate 23 Erythrasma showing typical coral fluorescence under Wood's light, described on page 120.

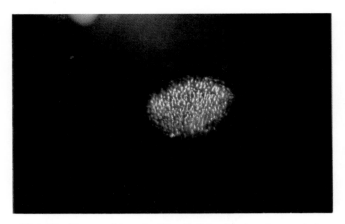

Plate 24 Tinea capitis under Wood's light showing characteristic blue-green fluorescence.

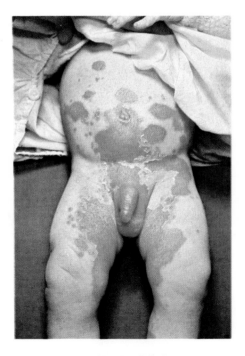

Plate 25 Candidiasis.

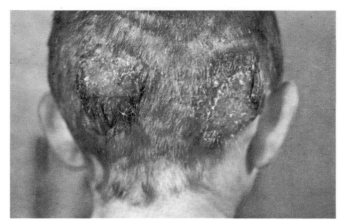

Plate 26   Kerion ringworm.

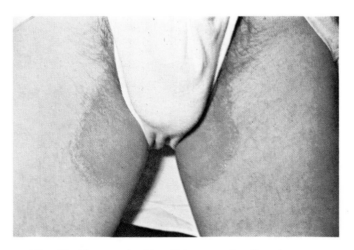

Plate 27   Tinea cruris with well demarcated scaling edge.

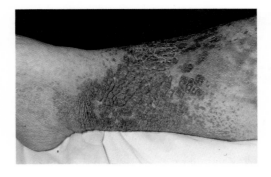

Plate 28 Gross diffuse gravitational scaling.

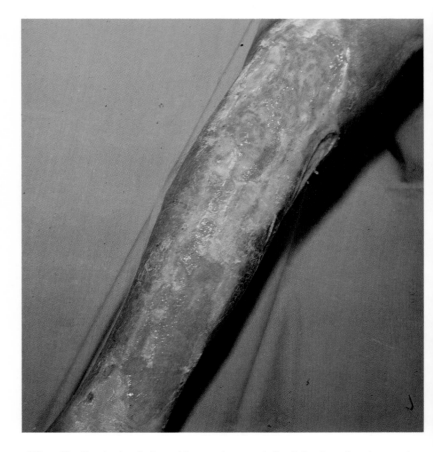

Plate 29 Gravitational ulcer with extensive excoriation following a knock at work. Healing was only possible after the patient had received compensation.

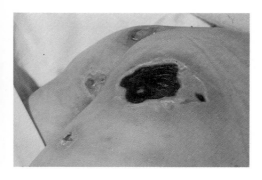

Plate 30 Pressure sores developing rapidly within a fortnight in a terminal illness.

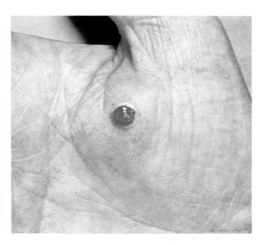

Plate 31 Pyogenic granuloma.

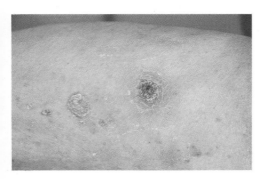

Plate 32 Solar keratoses showing as 'stuck on' lesions on an exposed area.

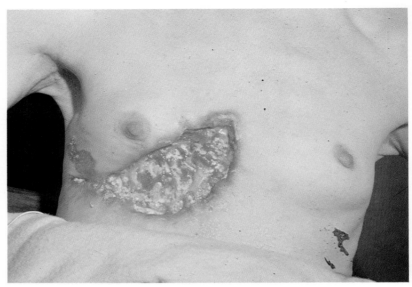

Plate 33 Neglected basal-cell carcinoma showing slow but relentless growth over a 25-year period.

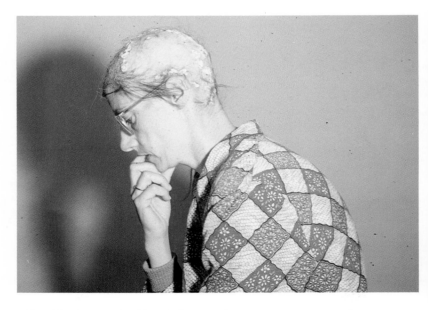

Plate 34 An example of favus infection before griseofulvin had been discovered. Stress may precipitate or worsen skin affections. On the other hand the presence of a physical skin disease may greatly distress the patient.

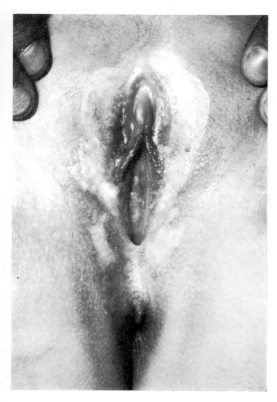

Fig. 43 Lichen sclerosus et atrophicus showing white infiltrated areas.

diseases of the Hodgkins-leukaemia group are described briefly on page 176.

Senile pruritus in an old person can denote stress if it follows within a few days of an upsetting event. More commonly it is due to long, hot baths and the excessive use of soaps. It may, however, be the first sign of internal malignancy and the relevant examinations and tests should be carried out as described in Chapter 9. Cimetidine, which is a histamine (H2) antagonist, sometimes helps to relieve itching. Symptomatic topical treatment is with emollient baths, corticosteroid creams, or a menthol, phenol and calamine lotion.

Purpura can occur in anaemia, leukaemia, Vitamin C deficiency and drug rashes. The lesions are petechial.

Internal malignancies

There are many dermatological manifestations of internal malignancy.

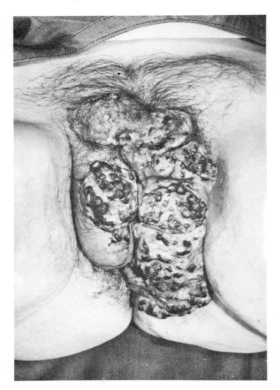

Fig. 44 Neglected lichen sclerosus et atrophicus developing leukoplakia and ultimately extensive squamous-cell carcinoma.

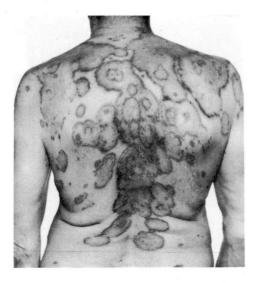

Fig. 45 Gyrate erythema from carcinoma of the bronchus.

A typical skin rash developing at unusual times or sites may give the first warning. Prurigo with undue pigmentation is an example. Pruritus and purpura from malignancy have already been mentioned. There are other rarities such as acanthosis nigracans, acquired ichthyosis, gyrate erythemas (Fig. 45) and malignant down.

Dermatomyositis

Dermatomyositis in older people is usually due to internal malignancy. Even a small primary growth can be responsible; there is a vigorous immunological attempt to control it, the skin and muscle being inadvertently attacked:

> The erythematous rash on the eyelids and backs of her hands was discussed at the dermatological meeting. She was presented for confirmation of the diagnosis of dermatomyositis on account of being perfectly fit, only 44 and full examination and tests giving normal results. 'Keep on looking,' was the advice. No change occurred for a year but then she began to develop muscle weakness. Palpation and special x-ray examination of breasts was normal. Three months later secondary deposits appeared in the neck, but the primary in the breast was barely palpable. She was dead within half a year.

Chapter 11. Granulomata including syphilis

A granuloma is a focal lesion caused by specific imflammatory cells or their degeneration products. The cellular reaction can be due either to chemical and physical agents or to certain infections. Most are fairly rare in Great Britain. This chapter covers granulomas of the skin caused by infections. The type and effectiveness of this cellular response depends on the patient's immunological ability to localise the infection as a granuloma. In a primary infection there are many organisms and little initial immunological response; when the infection is under control there is a good cellular response with a great reduction in the number of organisms.

Leprosy

Leprosy is a good example where the form that the illness takes depends upon the degree of host resistance by cell-mediated immunity. If the resistance is high the tuberculoid form occurs as either dry, scaly, asymmetrical areas (Figs. 46, 47), or as well-defined erythematous-edged, infiltrated plaques. Both have reduced pigmentation and cutaneous sensation and the lesions are rarely infectious. Conversely, if the host resistance is low the lepromatous form occurs as small, smooth-surfaced erythematous macules, often with increasing infiltration to form nodules and plaques, especially on the face and pinnae. These lesions can be infectious.

The larger nerves become palpable when involved. Enlargement of the ulnar nerve can be observed at the elbow, the peroneal nerve in the leg, and the great auricular nerve where it crosses the jaw. Decreased function may result in ulnar palsy or foot-drop respectively. Late in the illness a severe polyneuritis may develop.

Leprosy is due to an acid-fast bacillus, *Mycobacterium leprae*, similar to the one that causes tuberculosis. It is an illness transmitted by contact and by droplets from the upper respiratory tract, and should be considered in the differential diagnosis of any unusual rash which appears

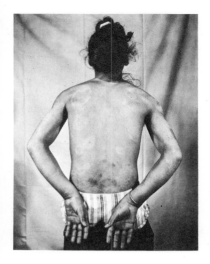

Fig. 46 Tuberculoid leprosy showing depigmented slightly scaly infiltrated areas on the back. The patient was born in India.

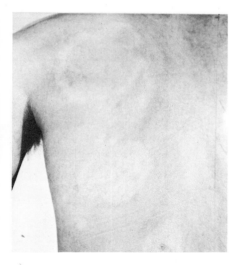

Fig. 47 Tuberculoid leprosy, a closer view of the lesions. The patches were anaesthetic.

within 2–7 years of being in tropical or subtropical climates. The name is descriptive, 'lepra' meaning 'scaly patch'.

Diagnosis is confirmed by biopsy, the bacilli being easily visible in the more lepromatous lesions but increasingly difficult to see in the more tuberculoid. Treatment is usually by oral dapsone, a sulphone, for a period of 2–4 years. The provision of a nutritious diet is also important. Advice on the care of anaesthetic areas is often given by the nurse. The patient must learn to strictly discipline himself to be very careful with objects that are sharp or hot, so that he does not harm himself. Movement can sometimes be effectively restored in a paralysed limb by tendon transplant operations, followed by rehabilitation; the patient has to learn that contraction of certain muscles causes different movements than before the operation.

Erythema nodosum is a clinical condition occasionally due to leprosy. Tender, red, smooth nodules appear usually on the shins. There is often associated pyrexia and joint symptoms. Erythema nodosum (Plate 21) is more commonly produced by streptococcal infections, sulphonamide reactions, tuberculosis or sarcoidosis.

Tuberculosis

Tuberculosis is a condition not only of the lungs and viscera but also of the skin. Infection with the acid-fast bacillus *Mycobacterium tuberculosis* results in granulomata; histologically these contain typical Langhans' giant cells and often central necrosis called caseation. Both human and cattle tuberculosis are now less prevalent in Britain because of effective chemotherapy and immunisation.

Primary tuberculosis of the skin occurs at the point of entry in a non-immune person as small persistent sores with local lymphadenopathy, rather similar to a BCG reaction (attenuated bovine bacillus used for immunisation against the disease). The sores may develop into painful ulcers with undermined edges. In a person who is immune to tuberculosis as a result of prior infection or immunisation, warty plaques occur at the point of entry. These used to be seen in slaughterhouse or post-mortem workers following a cut while handling the infected material.

Lupus vulgaris

Lupus vulgaris is due to secondary infection of the skin from tuberculosis elsewhere, usually via the lymphatics, and often from the neckglands or chest. The lesions are not infectious, only a few bacilli being contained by a good cellular response. Macroscopically, the lesions have a characteristic 'apple jelly' colour, best seen through a glass pressed firmly on the surface of the lesion. The diagnosis is confirmed by biopsy. Treatment is by specific chemotherapeutic agents, continuing for at least half a year after the lesion has slowly healed by scarring.

Sarcoidosis

Sarcoidosis of the skin looks similar to lupus vulgaris except that it is more plum coloured and not as scaly. There are also some differences in the histology. The cause is not yet fully established. Unlike lupus vulgaris the Mantoux test for tuberculosis is invariably negative. The Kveim test, however, is positive; the antigen, usually made from sterilised sarcoid spleen, is injected intradermally with the bevel of the needle uppermost. A ballpoint pen is used to mark the area, and the patient instructed to repeat the marking every few days. The area is biopsied after about 2 months, but earlier if a sarcoid nodule has developed. The test is positive if sarcoid granulomas are seen on histology.

Leishmaniasis

Cutaneous Leishmaniasis, also known as oriental sore, in the later stages may look like sarcoid or lupus vulgaris; earlier it may present as an active localised area of inflammation. The infection is transmitted by a tropical sandfly and therefore occurs on exposed areas of skin. It can be identified histologically by the presence of Leishman-Donovan bodies.

Syphilis

Syphilis is uncommon in Great Britain except amongst practising male homosexuals or in the type of shifting population found, for example, around ports. It is a granulomatous systemic condition caused by infection with the spirochaete *Treponema pallidum*.

The primary lesions are called chancres. They appear at the point of infection as indurated rubbery papules, erosions or ulcers, usually with a scant exudate. There is usually very little pain, which is the main reason why a quarter of all cases are overlooked, especially when the cervix is affected. The majority of lesions occur on the anogenital organs of both sexes, 95% of syphilis being sexually transmitted. The incubation time is between 2 and 5 weeks. About a week after the development of the primary lesion there is a localised lymphadenopathy usually associated with general malaise.

If untreated, primary syphilis will progress to secondary syphilis at 3–6 months after contact. This can affect the nervous system, eyes, bones and viscera. There is a general malaise including a temperature, headache and generalised lymphadenopathy. In three-quarters of cases a non-specific, varied and widespread rash is present. This rarely itches and is quite unlike the primary chancre which is by now healing or healed. It is commonly composed of delicate rose coloured macules, often difficult to see except in daylight. The lesions can also be maculo-papular or papular in nature, in which case they tend to be more coppery in colour.

In flexural areas the lesions become heaped up into moist, shiny, flat, fleshy plaques or nodules called condylomata lata. These occur especially in the anogenital, submammary and axillary regions, but also at the angles of the mouth and between fingers and toes. In the mouth, greyishwhite mucous patches and snailtrack ulcers may occur. As in all secondary syphilitic lesions, infection of contacts is a distinct possibility. This must be borne in mind whilst nursing or examining patients before treatment has started; gloves should always be worn. The secondary stage lasts for up to 2 years, during which patchy hair loss from the scalp, beard and eyebrows may occur. Untreated, secondary syphilis will progress to tertiary syphilis.

The granuloma of tertiary syphilis is called a gumma. The lesions appear as well-defined reddish nodules up to 1 cm in diameter, which break down to form discrete, punched-out ulcers with a sloughing base. The local necrotic change is brought about by damage to small arterioles. Alternatively, the lesions may be of varied shape with a well-defined edge, similar to lupus vulgaris. These all heal leaving scar tissue:

> She had an angular look, and her gaze was stern as one accustomed to handling people. Two years previously a painless nodular lesion had developed over her left shoulder. Part of it had healed leaving tissue paper scarring, but it was still unsightly and she sought advice. The young registrar queried a diagnosis of lupus vulgaris, but the consultant shook his head—'Very unusual for it to develop at the age of 60, and the onset of scarring is far too quick; it is a healing gumma—What is your occupation?' 'I am retired now, but we billeted soldiers 10 years ago. I was a landlady.'

However, much more important in tertiary syphilis are the systemic changes in the cardiovascular and central nervous systems, and viscera These include heart damage, aortic aneurysms, and infection of the nervous tissue causing tabes dorsalis or general paralysis of the insane. By this stage treponemes are rarely found and sufferers are not infectious.

Routine antenatal serology has dramatically reduced the incidence of congenital syphilis which occurs following transplacental passage of the treponemes. In earlier times abortion, systemic illness, and neonatal deaths were often caused by this condition.

Until the diagnosis is confirmed, the synonym 'Lues' should be used; the word 'syphilis' is highly emotive because of the obvious implications of how it is contracted. During the primary stage, discharge from a lesion is examined for treponemes by dark-ground illumination microscopy. In the secondary stage this is also possible from the condylomata, but spirochaetes are not usually found in the tertiary stage.

The Wasserman reaction (WR) is a useful screening test but false negatives may occasionally occur late in the tertiary stages. False positives occur with yaws and sometimes with leprosy, malaria and glandular fever. More specific tests are therefore required with all positive results.

The demonstration of antibodies to the organism is a much more expensive but effective method. Currently used are the treponemal immobilisation test (TPI), and the fluorescent treponemal antibody test (FTA). While being far more accurate than the WR, they also give an indication of the body's immunological response to the infection; if a patient with primary syphilis defaults from treatment the prognosis is far worse if he is seronegative rather than seropositive. A worse prognosis also occurs following inadequate antibiotic therapy given inadvertently when a primary lesion is misdiagnosed as a boil or a similar pyogenic infection.

In North America and Britain the treatment of syphilis is now usually undertaken by the venereologist. Massive doses of aqueous procaine penicillin, such as 1–2 mega units, are given as daily intramuscular injections for up to 10 days in the early stages, and for up to 3 weeks in the later stages of syphilis. Tracing the origin of the infection and all contacts is very important. However, care is needed as otherwise there can be great family and psychological upset.

Health education plays a preventive role. The use of the condom is encouraged; it was invented as a preventive barrier against infection, not conception! Education also draws the public's attention to the early signs and symptoms of venereal disease, and from where accurate diagnosis and treatment can be obtained under conditions of strict confidentiality. Fortunately, the old sailor stamping his 'tabetic two-step' down the road to the docks is a thing of the past, but not to be forgotten.

Chapter 12. Infections—bacterial, fungal and viral

Infections occur when the skin defences fail or the patient's susceptibility is increased. They also occur when the organisms are present in overwhelming numbers or when they have increased in virulence.

The normal skin provides a chemical and physical barrier against the majority of organisms. The fatty acids in sebum are bacteriostatic and fungistatic; sweat is bactericidal and together with desiccation will destroy most pathogens. The horny layer is a physical barrier, but is relatively susceptible to alkalis, solvents or keratolytics, and can also be breached by injury. Any skin lesion which weakens the physical barrier, such as psoriasis, eczema or dermatitis, increases the chance of penetration, especially if there is moisture and trauma. Systemic and local steroids also increase the chance of infection by interfering with the body's immunological defence mechanisms.

The skin's normal response to invasion is to release histamine and other related substances. These increase tissue perfusion and enable inflammatory cells to congregate more quickly. Later, specific antibodies are produced against the invading organisms. The treatment of skin infection is aimed at helping the skin to heal itself. As dry skin is more resistant it is important to keep the surfaces cool; the exception is when the tissue is also affected by arteriosclerotic disease, where vasoconstriction should be avoided. When dressings are required they must be non-occlusive in nature. The use of light clothing will reduce any trauma from friction. Above all, any local treatments must be non-toxic to the skin and not interfere with normal defence mechanisms.

Granulomatous lesions are caused by specific organisms and have been dealt with in the last chapter. This chapter covers the common organisms which are usually present on our skins for most of the time. These fall into three groups: bacteria, fungi and viruses.

Bacterial infections

Staphylococci are Gram-positive bacteria which form a large percentage of man's commensal flora and account for the majority of his acute and chronic suppurative lesions. They are only pathogenic when present in large numbers. The most virulent and therefore important strain is called *Staphylococcus pyogenes*. It is usually resistant to penicillin therapy, but antibiotics are not normally required anyway unless the lesions become widespread, excessively large, or if there is systemic infection.

The bacteria are usually spread by asymptomatic carriers, especially hospital staff, in their anterior nasal cavities and on their perineum and skin. Contacts should always be examined therefore, swabs being taken for culture and sensitivity, and treatment carried out as required on the other members of the family or institution. Ultraviolet light is often useful in reducing the numbers of skin pathogens. Antiseptic baths will also reduce the skin reservoir of organisms. A suitable one can be prepared by dissolving approximately 4 teaspoonfuls of potassium permanganate crystals in a bowl of hot water, which solution is then added to the full bath; this minimises staining, which can be removed by dilute oxalic acid, unfortunately along with some of the glaze! Smaller amounts are required for foot baths or Sitz baths which are very useful for symptomatic relief of weeping areas; chlorhexidine 0.02% in water is an alternative but more expensive preparation and does not stain.

Twice-daily applications should be made of dibromopropamidine (Brulidine) or chlorhexidine creams to the nares and perineum. Children who are carriers should be kept well away from babies or from school until swabs show that they have been cleared.

The infected lesions also need treatment to reduce the number of organisms present. If dibromopropamidine or chlorhexidine creams do not clear them, then the dyes should be used; crystal violet 0.5% in water is the most effective and has the added advantage of drying an exudative area, further reducing the infection. It hardly ever produces a sensitivity dermatitis.

Dyes are not effective against Gram-negative infections, as can be seen from Fig. 76. These organisms, which include pseudomonas and proteus, can also cause skin infections and are carried in the gut. Patients should therefore be encouraged to wash their hands thoroughly with soap and water after toilet. These Gram-negative infections should be treated with silver nitrate 0.5% cream or lotion, as detailed for leg ulcers from page 149. Polynoxylin powder is a less effective preparation but is cleaner and easier to use.

114   *Chapter 12*

Furunculosis

Furunculosis (boils) are an invasion of the sebaceous glands and hair
follicles, usually by a pathogenic staphylococcus, when there is reduced
local or general resistance to infection. They usually occur at sites of
maceration and recurrent trauma such as chafing and scratching. They
are more common in diabetes, seborrhoea and immunologically deficient patients. It is important to look for these underlying causes.
Furunculosis usually occurs after puberty and may be single or multiple.
Large multiple lesions are called carbuncles. Recurrent boils require
treatment for 2 months after the last lesion has cleared, so that the
residual number of organisms on the skin can be reduced in number.
Carriers within the family must of course also be treated. It is unusual
for this staphylococcus to cause impetigo, a condition which will be
described later.

Hydradenitis suppurativa

Hydradenitis suppurativa (axillary boils) is an infection of the apocrine
glands in the axilla, usually by a pathogenic staphylococcus. It can also
occur in the glands of the groins. The resulting fibrosis and scarring can
be minimised by the early topical application of clioquinol. If the condition becomes extensive, systemic and local antibiotics as well as surgical
drainage may be needed. The cells of the cyst wall may then require
destruction by diathermy, or by the introduction of phenol on the end
of a sharp implement as described on page 182.

Folliculitis

Folliculitis is an inflammation of the hair follicle. It is more common
in seborrhoeic patients and may also occur following the use of crude
coal tar, occlusive steroid therapy, or contact with industrial oils
followed by recurrent trauma.

Infectious dermatitis

Infectious dermatitis is an exuding eczematous reaction around cracks,
and is usually due to a staphylococcal infection. Common sites include
the angles of the mouth and eyes, behind the ears and in the anal cleft.
Local spread can be very rapid. Topical steroids are required in addition to the usual anti-infective therapy.

Toxic epidermal necrolysis

Toxic epidermal necrolysis in children (Lyell-Ritter's disease) is the result of a toxin produced by specific strains of staphylococci. It is a serious condition in which there is a widespread shedding of the epidermis, and requires the local and usually systemic use of antibiotics. A similar condition is seen in adults but this is caused by drugs.

Paronychia of the newborn

Paronychia of the newborn is due to *Staphylococcus pyogenes* and requires only local treatment. The same bacteria are responsible for a large proportion of impetigo cases of all ages.

Impetigo

Impetigo is usually a primary condition, but can also be secondary to eczema, dermatitis, psoriasis, or from scratching due to scabies, pediculosis capitis or papular urticaria. The face is the commonest area to be affected (Fig. 48). The initial small erythematous area enlarges

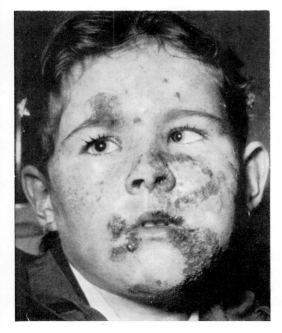

Fig. 48 Impetigo showing typical crusted localised lesions.

rapidly into a spreading vesicle which bursts and forms a scab. When the scalp is involved, there is matting of the hair; this distinguishes it from ringworm. As with all the other infections, the source should be found wherever possible. Relative isolation of the patient is necessary to prevent cross-infection, and must be stringent if any babies are in close proximity. Towels, sponges, brushes and combs should not be shared, and close contact avoided. Impetigo of the newborn is rare. It usually blisters and can be extensive or even fatal unless treated by antibiotics. While the sensitivity of the organism is being obtained, erythromycin should be given internally and sodium fucidate ointment used locally. The old name for the condition was pemphigus neonatorum which was a notifiable disease. Nasal and perineal swabs should be taken from those attending the baby in order to identify any carriers.

The lesions of impetigo due to streptococcal infections are less localised and more scabbed. Treatment with dibromopropamidine cream twice daily is usually quickly effective, but with severe infection it may be necessary to change to neomycin cream and give systemic penicillin in addition.

Streptococci are also Gram-positive cocci, and make up a large proportion of the normal bacterial flora, especially of the respiratory and alimentary tracts. *Streptococcus faecalis* is the most common, but is usually not pathogenic. The most virulent strain is called *Streptococcus pyogenes* or haemolytic streptococcus. Whereas the staphylococci tend to wall themselves off into abscesses, streptococci tend to spread through the tissues. They are common secondary invaders, resulting in an inflammatory halo around existing more purulent lesions, with red streaks of lymphangitis and tender local lymphadenopathy. A rare but potentially lethal glomerulonephritis may occur as the result of an immune reaction; there appears to be an antigenic similarity between the infecting organism and certain renal tissues. Because of this, penicillin V must be used whenever a haemolytic streptococcal infection is suspected, the organism virtually always being sensitive.

Cellulitis

Cellulitis is an inflammation of the skin and the subcutaneous tissues, usually due to a streptococcus. Infection with the more pathogenic streptococcus causes the condition called *erysipelas* where there is more systemic change. This is an acute febrile illness with a very rapid onset in which rigors often occur. As the management and treatment of both conditions are similar they are described together.

The haemolytic streptococcus usually gains access through a minute crack which has occurred as the result of trauma. On the face this is usually at the corner of the mouth or ear, whereas on the lower limbs it is from between the toes as the result of trauma or fungal infection. There is a rapidly spreading area of erythema and oedema, typically with advancing red streaks of lymphangitis. In the absence of a history of penicillin allergy, the antibiotic should immediately be given by injection. The course can be completed by mouth as soon as improvement is noted. Swabs should be taken initially to confirm the diagnosis. Topical application of sodium fucidate, neomycin or crystal violet is needed. Recurrent attacks are common and may damage the lymphatics causing lymphoedema which, in the case of a leg, may require permanent elastic support.

Erysipeloid

Erysipeloid is a similar but much less pathogenic specific local infection contracted by handlers of uncooked shellfish, fish, meat or poultry. There is a more purple erythema with the well-defined, raised, spreading edge but with little systemic upset. The organism is virtually always sensitive to penicillin.

Erythrasma

Erythrasma is a circumscribed infection of the groins, axillae, or toe clefts, more common but similar in nature to a low-grade fungal infection (Plate 22). It is caused by a specific Gram-positive bacillus called *Corynebacterium minutissimum*. The coral fluorescence of erythrasma (Plate 23), when viewed under Wood's lamp (described later), is probably its main diagnostic feature. Unlike other fungi it responds to systemic antibiotics such as erythromycin or tetracycline. Local treatment is as for fungi.

Intertrigo

Intertrigo due to low-grade infection has already been described in the section on seborrhoeic dermatitis. More virulent infections in flexural areas can cause erosions and considerable soreness. Frequent applications of gauze moistened with antiseptic solutions are needed. Swabs should be taken and appropriate systemic antibiotics given if improvement is not satisfactory. A urine test for sugar is mandatory as with all infections. Intertrigo should not be confused with flexural psoriasis

(Plate 3), which is well demarcated, salmon coloured and has typical lesions elsewhere.

Fungal infections

Mycoses are diseases caused by fungal infections. This group includes the true fungi, the yeasts, and the yeast-like fungi.

Pityriasis versicolor

Pityriasis versicolor is a superficial skin infection by the specific yeast-like fungus called *Malassezia furfur*. In the warmer climates this occurs predominantly as light brown, faintly scaling, macular lesions, usually on the trunk and shoulders of young adults. Conversely in the dark-skinned races, and also in the 'whites' after sunbathing, the lesions appear as depigmented areas of scaling. Scrapings show fungus filaments (mycelia). Selenium sulphide (available as a shampoo called Selsun) should be applied at weekly intervals to the lesions for 3 weeks. Alternatively econazole cream should be applied twice daily for 2 weeks.

Candida albicans

Candida albicans is another yeast-like fungus and is carried in the gut of about 1 in 5 individuals as a commensal organism. When present in quantity it causes an infection called moniliasis or candidiasis. This occurs in the weak and debilitated, and very young and very old, the immunodeficient and in diabetics. Overgrowth of yeasts and clostridia also follows antibiotic therapy; this is because these organisms are resistant but most of the other commensals are sensitive, leaving a space which they then fill to restore the ecological balance. This over-growth is the main cause of the antibiotic diarrhoea from wide spectrum antibiotics; it can usually be prevented by natural yoghurt, which contains non-pathogenic lactobacilli, taken between the antibiotic doses. A carton per day is usually sufficient.

Oral infection is called 'thrush', with spreading 'milk spots', patches and plaques, which can be removed by scraping to reveal erythematous areas. Vaginal infection results in similar patches, plus a thick white curd-like discharge. Vulvitis and balanitis may also occur. Candidal intertrigo is typically a glazed erythematous area (Plate 25) surrounded by vesicles or pustules. Fresh scales or the roof of a vesicle should be sent for examination wherever possible before treatment is commenced, which should be with pessaries, tablets or cream containing nystatin, econazole, clotrimazole, miconazole or amphotericin B. Aqueous crystal violet or magenta paint are often more effective but colourful! Resistant oral thrush responds best to the sucking of nystatin pessaries which are unfortunately bitter; do not use the effervescent variety!

Chronic paronychia

Chronic paronychia usually follows trauma or prolonged immersion in water or beer, and is commonly found in domestic workers and barmaids. The base of the nail becomes inflamed like an inflated pillow and pus can often be expressed (Fig. 49); this procedure should only take place when a swab is required, as any rubbing or squeezing of the lesions interferes with healing. *Candida* is almost invariably the organism involved. When the inflammation is acute, swabs often show a secondary infection with *Staphylococcus pyogenes*, and in these cases an appropriate antibiotic such as erythromycin should be given.

General advice includes keeping the areas warm and dry. When the fingernails are affected it is important either to avoid wet work or to wear rubber or plastic gloves over cotton ones. The cotton gloves should be kept dry by using several pairs in rotation. If the toes are

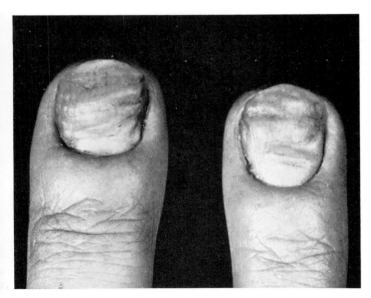

Fig. 49   Chronic paronychia showing inflammation of nail base and deformity of nails.

affected cotton socks and open sandals should be worn. Occasionally washing the area is allowed provided that the nail fold is first protected with nystatin ointment. This application should be repeated afterwards and the treatment continued at least twice daily until the cuticle has entirely regrown. Econazole cream is a really effective alternative treatment provided the area can be kept dry. Resistant cases may need a course of superficial X-ray treatment, described on page 194, or even the following regime:

1   First thing in the morning magenta paint or crystal violet 0.5% in 70% spirit should be applied to the affected nail folds.
2   When this has dried the folds should be sealed with acrylic resin. The patient should not undertake morning toilet washing until the seal has dried. The seal should be reapplied during the daytime as necessary. When doing any heavy washing it is better to wear a rubber glove on top of the seal to prevent it from breaking.
3   Last thing at night (after toilet washing has been completed) the acrylic resin should be removed with acetone or nail-varnish remover.
4   A further application of the dye should then be made. The treatment should be continued until the cuticle has entirely regrown.

Ringworm

Ringworm is a group of conditions caused by infection with fungi. It is more common in close communities, being transmitted via floors and towels, in showers and swimming baths, as well as by direct contact. The chance of infection is also increased by warmth, moisture and recurrent trauma or chafing such as occurs on the feet, axillae and in the groins. The clinical conditions can each be caused by different organisms, of which only the common ones will be described. Confirmatory diagnosis is by microscopy and culture, as detailed on page 189.

Diagnosis with Wood's lamp. The Wood's lamp has aided the diagnosis and differentiation of some fungi. This is an ultraviolet lamp with a filter of cobalt and nickel glass that removes the visible light and is similar to those used in discotheques. Certain organisms and materials convert the ultraviolet light into visible light, which appears as a fluorescence when viewed in a darkened room. *Microsporon audouinii* and *M. canis* give off a brilliant green fluorescence (Plate 24), while favus (*Trichophyton schoenleinii*) appears as a paler yellow-green. Pityriasis versicolor sometimes looks a dirty yellow-brown, whereas erythrasma is a bright coral pink (Plate 23). All the other important organisms do not fluoresce.

Tinea capitis presents as an irregular-shaped alopecia, with scalp changes that can range from a slight scaling and erythema to a severe pustular reaction. The organisms penetrate the hair follicles and the hairs become brittle, breaking off just above the scalp. The rare human form is due to *Microsporon audouinii*, whereas the commoner microsporon canis is caught from cats and dogs. Dry scaling areas with broken hairs can be seen. Permanent alopecia does not occur if early and adequate treatment is given. More inflammation is produced by the bovine cattle ringworm called *Trichophyton verrucosum*, which affects farming families and slaughter-house men. Typically there are single or multiple boggy, heaped up, painless, granulomatous domes called kerion (Plate 26), often covered by sterile pustules. Treatment, or the natural development of immunity, ultimately results in resolution but some alopecia is permanent. All cattle, pets and rodents may also carry *trichophyton mentagraphytes* which can produce a similar clinical picture.

Secondary infection by staphylococci often considerably aggravates an animal ringworm on a hairy area. Staphylococci are fortunately sensitive to econazole, which is also effective against the fungi.

Favus causes a specific tinea capitis, a rare form of scalp ringworm with cup-shaped adherent yellow crusts and a 'mousey' odour. If untreated it will progress to a permanently scarring alopecia (Plate 34).

Tinea corporis is due to infection of the skin with any of the abovementioned fungi. It is of interest that the non-human varieties tend to cause more inflammatory reaction as the fungi are not adapted to living on their human hosts. A typical ringed appearance is produced with a scaling, raised, expanding, erythematous edge surrounding a quiescent centre. Cattle ringworm can be caught from fences or gates against which infected cattle have rubbed, in which case it usually affects the wrists.

Tinea cruris, also known as Dhobie itch, is ringworm of the groins and is usually caused by *Epidermophyton floccosum*. There is a similarly demarcated scaling edge but the central scaling is fine. The lesions can extend to the thighs and trunk. Tinea cruris can also be produced by the types of fungi which affect the feet, which can be spread by scratching. Both sites should therefore always be examined and treated accordingly.

Tinea pedis (athlete's foot) is the commonest fungal infection and is usually produced by *Trichophyton interdigitale*. This is probably the human counterpart of *T. mentagrophytes*, which therefore produces less host reaction. *Epidermophyton floccosum* is also common. The diagnosis should be suspected in anyone with unilateral scaling and cracks between the toes and can be confirmed by scrapings from the scaling margin. *Trichophyton rubrum* requires a special mention as the clinical picture is slightly different. It has adapted to human infection, and therefore produces less inflammatory reaction and is more difficult to eradicate. There is sodden, 'blotting-paper' skin in the little-toe cleft and sometimes a chronic unilateral dry scaling of the palms, buttocks or lower legs (Fig. 50a, b, d).

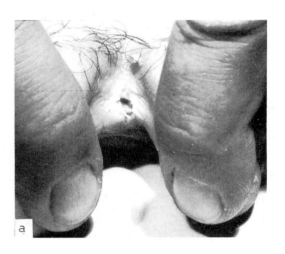

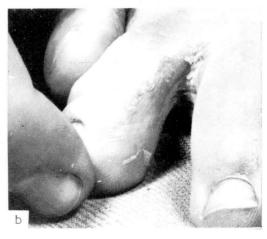

Fig. 50a–d
Trichophyton rubrum
infection, showing
maceration, cracking
and peeling (a & b),

Tinea pedis can also be caused by *Trichophyton tonsurans* and *T. violaceum*. These are rare in Great Britain but are important pathogens abroad. Together with *Trichophyton rubrum* they are notorious for infecting nails, causing off-white opaque areas which become more powdery and hyperkeratotic as the condition progresses. The presence of longitudinal columns of altered nail is diagnostic (Fig. 50c). The condition is initially unilateral which distinguishes it from psoriatic changes, as well as by the absence of pits or the rash elsewhere. Microscopy and culture of nail clippings are required to confirm the diagnosis, and should be carried out as outlined on page 189.

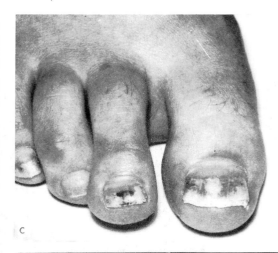

(c) longitudinal columns of nail infection

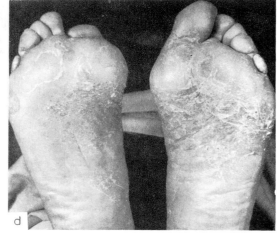

(d) dry scaling.

Treatment of fungal infections

Treatment of fungus infections is mainly undertaken with local applications, but as infection of the actual nail only responds to the antifungal antibiotic griseofulvin, this drug will be described first. It is normally given in a single daily dose after the main meal as fat aids its absorption, but divided doses may be needed if there is gastrointestinal upset. The normal adult dose is 500 mg daily. It is deposited in newly formed keratin and this prevents further invasion by the fungus. Fingernails take half a year to grow out and toenails up to 2 years, particularly in the aged. The drug has therefore to be continued regularly for these periods if the fungus is to be eradicated. Failure is usually due to low blood levels from poor absorption of the drug. Alternatively, if only a few toenails are affected they can be removed under ring-block or general anaesthesia. This procedure reduces the griseofulvin treatment to 1 month before and 1 month after the operation. Local treatment after surgery is by application of griseofulvin powder daily for a week and then benzoic acid compound ointment until the nail has regrown. It is mandatory that any fungus infection of the toe clefts is eradicated at the same time by the local treatments to be described, otherwise re-infection will take place. *Trichophyton rubrum* infections of the skin do not heal without combined external and internal therapy. Regular follow-up is needed to make sure that this is carried out.

Griseofulvin has revolutionised the treatment of scalp and animal ringworm. A 3-week course is usually adequate providing that topical fungicides are used in addition. It should be remembered that griseofulvin is not effective against yeasts such as candida, or in the treatment of pityriasis versicolor or erythrasma.

Local applications are the mainstay in the treatment of ringworm of the skin. Many different preparations have been advocated. The more recently introduced creams containing econazole, miconazole or clotrimazole are effective and cosmetically acceptable, but are expensive and need to be applied twice daily. Benzoic acid compound ointment BPC (Whitfield's) has been used since the beginning of the century, and if applied daily is just as effective. Unless diluted it is unfortunately too irritant to be used on the face, axillary, submammary or anogenital regions. In these areas daily applications of magenta paint BPC (Castellani's) is cheap and effective. Treatment should always be continued for at least a fortnight after clearance, and should be followed by fungicidal dusting powders such as clotrimazole or tolnaftate for a further 2 months. This is again to prevent reinfection. These periods should be doubled in *Trichophyton rubrum* infections, in which it is sometimes necessary to use the benzoic acid compound ointment at twice its normal strength in order to eradicate the infection.

Preventing the spread of infection or reinfection requires personal towels, sponges, face cloths, clothing and shoes. Floors should be thoroughly cleaned and disinfected. Slippers or shoes should have a swab soaked in 15% formalin placed in them in a confined space for 1 day, followed by exposure to the open air for at least 2 days to let it evaporate.

Ringworm is occasionally confused in children with a localised degenerative collagen disease called granuloma annulare. This condition does not scale and has no spreading edge. It is composed of annular smooth granulomatous areas. Treatment is only needed for cosmetic reasons, and should then be with strong steroids suitably localised.

Dermatitis of the feet can also be confused with tinea pedis; the ringworm primarily affects the skin between the toes but may extend to involve the adjacent skin. In dermatitis the backs of the toes and feet are primarily affected, as has been discussed earlier.

Hyperidrosis is a condition where there is excessive sweating. When present on the soles it is often misdiagnosed as tinea pedis. There is moistness and maceration of the toes and clefts and the weight-bearing area of the soles, all having a characteristic livid erythematous colour. It should be treated with formaldehyde 3% soaks for 10 minutes each evening, or alternatively with localised glutaraldehyde 10% solution on alternate evenings. When hyperidrosis involves the axilla, aluminium chloride hexahydrate 20% in absolute alcohol can be used. This must be applied to the dried, unwashed, hairy area, otherwise there can be an excessive reaction. Application should be nightly for a week, and then less frequently as sweating diminishes. The preparation should be washed off the following morning. Irritation caused by the treatment can be controlled by applying hydrocortisone cream.

Viral infections

Virus infections differ from those caused by bacteria and fungi in that the organisms actually enter into the host cells to alter their structure and function.

Pityriasis rosea

Pityriasis rosea is believed to be viral in origin. Attacks are commoner in the spring and young people are usually affected. Fine scaling erythematous lesions affect the trunk and proximal ends of the limbs about a week after the development of a larger lesion, known as a 'herald spot'. The lesions follow the lines of the ribs and continue on the adjacent parts of the limbs, taking about 6 weeks to clear. Treatment is just to allay irritation with an oral antihistamine and an intermediate strength topical steroid.

Herpes simplex

Herpes simplex (cold sores) is an infection with a specific herpes virus. Characteristically there are burning crops of vesicles, usually around the mouth or genitalia, which progress into small ulcers that become crusted. The lesions resolve spontaneously after about 2 weeks. The primary infection occurs within the first 5 years of life, the virus remaining dormant in the local nerve ganglion. Reactivation of the virus is usually brought about by sunlight, a high fever, a menstrual period, or psychological pressure or upset. The virus often also affects the mucosa of the mouth as multiple aphthous ulcers, and occasionally the eyes as a conjunctivitis. The latter may develop into a keratitis and even dendritic ulcers which require specialist attention. Herpes simplex infection of an eczema sufferer has already been discussed on page 41.

Idoxuridine (IDU) is the mainstay of treatment, but is only effective if applied at the onset of the condition whilst the virus is still dividing. The IDU 5% in dimethyl sulphoxide should be applied 4 times a day to the skin for a period of only 4 days. IDU 0.1% solution is used for treatment of the eyes.

Recurrent attacks of herpes may be quite troublesome, and may even cause attacks of erythema multiforme of the hands, feet, lips and in the mouth. Antipyretics such as aspirin may prevent recurrences caused by fever or sunlight.

Herpes varicella

Herpes varicella (chicken pox) is due to another specific herpes virus and usually occurs during the first decade of life. It is a highly infectious but mild illness, with distinctive crops of vesicles affecting the trunk more than the face and limbs. The vesicles are each surrounded by a pink erythematous halo and progress to pustules and eventually scabs. The lesions are present at different stages of development as they appear in crops on successive days. Skin treatment should be aimed at preventing secondary infection in order to minimise scarring.

Herpes zoster

Herpes zoster (shingles) is caused by the reactivation of the same virus, and can occur after the second decade of life whenever there is a depressed host immunological response. Pain, which can be intense, usually precedes the appearance of the rash by about 3 days, and each episode is usually over within a fortnight. The lesions are grouped vesicles on an inflamed base (Fig. 51), similar to an extensive simplex

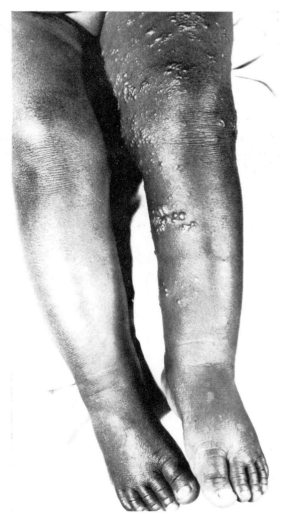

Fig. 51 Herpes zoster showing grouped vesicles.

infection, usually becoming haemorrhagic and eventually forming crusts. They follow the skin distribution of the affected nerve, and therefore do not cross the midline. The virus can affect any nerve, but especially involves those of the scalp, face and back. Resolution is usually complete, but the condition often results in permanent scarring. At the onset the condition should also be treated with IDU and later with topical applications against secondary bacterial infection as required. If lesions present after the first few days, painkillers and frequent application of calamine lotion should be given. Post-herpetic pain can be severe, and can persist for months or even years after the infection. It is poorly controlled by painkillers, and sometimes even requires surgical destruction of the ganglia as a last resort. Various combinations of phenothiazines, tricyclic antidepressants or anticonvulsants should always be tried beforehand. If the ophthalmic branch of the trigeminal nerve is involved, specialist attention may be required for treatment of any conjunctivitis, keratitis and also a form of glaucoma.

Variola

Variola (smallpox) is caused by a specific virus of a different type, a pox virus. The condition is highly infectious and often fatal. The lesions are similar to those of varicella, but are all at the same stage of development and tend to be more extensive on the face and periphery of the limbs. Treatment, as far as the skin is concerned, is to prevent secondary bacterial infection. Fortunately vaccination and health control have eradicated the virus, with the exception of cultures preserved in certain laboratories.

Molluscum contagiosum

Molluscum contagiosum are multiple, warty, dome-shaped skin nodules which are believed to be due to infection by another specific pox virus (Fig. 52). It is transferred by contact and is more common in children. The nodules are usually waxy pink and have an umbilicated centre. Spontaneous resolution takes place as immunity develops. Mothers who are anxious to actively treat their children should apply an antiseptic paint on the lesions daily. When destructive treatment is needed the white curd-like contents should be expressed. Alternatively it is less painful to prick the umbilicated centre with a sharpened applicator dipped in phenol. Cryotherapy, described on page 183, is a quicker alternative.

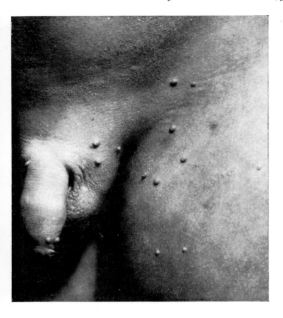

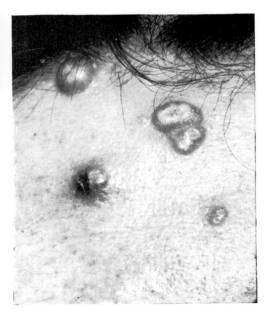

Figs. 52a & b
Molluscum
contagiosum.

Warts

Warts are caused by infection with a papovavirus, literally a member of the 'viruses of papilloma' group (Fig. 53). Warts can be single or multiple and often follow the line of an old scratch. They are usually round or oval and vary in size from 1 to 10 mm (Fig. 54). Although the surface may be smooth, as in plane warts, an excrescence of yellow brown and even black keratin is usually seen coming from the top of the lesion. Infection is from human contact and from communal floors and articles. The majority resolve spontaneously within 2 years as immunity to the virus develops. The treatment of warts, therefore, ranges from hypnosis and wart charming to the physical destruction of the lesions by chemicals or freezing. A good compromise is to use antiseptics to prevent further spread whilst natural immunity develops.

Plane warts occur mainly on the hands and face of young people. On the face they are best left alone, but if necessary salicylic acid 3% in aqueous cream can be used; caustics should obviously be kept well away from the eyes and chlorhexidine 0.5% in 70% spirit accurately applied twice daily.

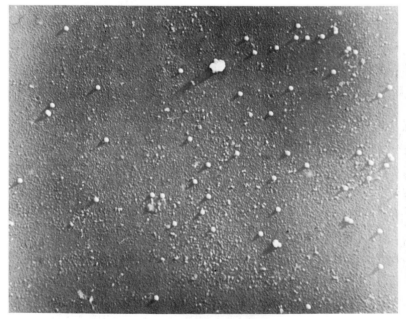

Fig. 53 Electronmicrograph of an extract of a plantar wart showing virus-like bodies, taken in 1950 before the cause had been proved.

Silver nitrate can be applied daily to warts of the fingers as an aqueous 1–3% solution or as a 'stick'. The silver turns the warts black. Formaldehyde and glutaraldehyde (Glutarol) solutions or salicylic acid colloidin BPC applied twice daily is an alternative. Salicylic acid is also available as an impregnated plaster, which is effective on warts of the fingers and plantar warts:

> Cut the salicylic acid 40% plaster accurately to fit the wart and keep in position with adhesive strapping. After 5–7 days the wart is sufficiently macerated for the top layers to be curetted away. This process should be repeated at 5–7-day intervals until the wart has gone. Cure depends mostly on the thorough removal of dead tissue.

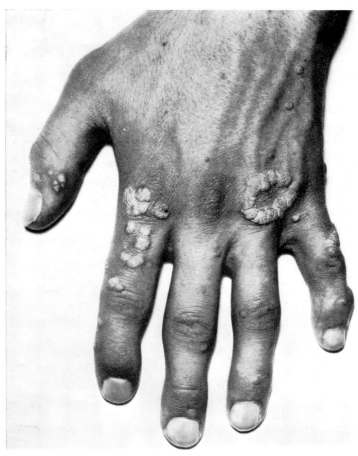

Fig. 54 Common warts.

Patients can carry out this removal with the blade of a pair of rounded scissors. Doctors or nurses should use a curette if available and apply liquefied phenol BP afterwards to assist the removal of dead tissue and virus particles. The treatment of warts at the base of the nail (periungual) is similar to the above, except that one single accurate application of monochloracetic acid should first be made to the wart and the salicylic acid plaster left in position for 3 days only. The development of secondary infection often cures a wart.

Plantar warts occur on the feet where the lesion is unable to proliferate above the surface of the skin due to pressure from weight bearing. They can be very painful. Mosaic warts are more numerous but superficial. They can all be treated as follows:

> The dead tissue and scales must first be removed each evening with the side of a blade of round-ended scissors. Then soak the wart-bearing portions of the sole of the foot for 15–20 minutes in formaldehyde 3% solution BP. The strength should be increased by 2% each fortnight (up to 9%) until the skin round the wart is dry and cracked. (Soft paraffin is needed to protect the more tender skin between the toes from the treatment.) The wart must not be placed in contact with the bottom of the dish containing the solution. Success usually depends on the patient carrying out the detailed treatment each evening. Patients may need assistance or encouragement in removing the dead tissue from the larger warts.

Condyloma accuminatum (soft warts) are moist and filiform, and occur in the anogenital region as they are often sexually transmitted; the actual site usually gives an indication of the source (Fig. 55). Twice-daily paintings with glutarldehyde should be used first. Resistant lesions may need local antimitotic treatments such as podophyllin 30% in acetone. These have to be applied very carefully using a cottonwool-tipped applicator, as otherwise severe inflammation and ulceration can occur. The surrounding skin should be powdered with talcum and after 6 hours washed with soap and warm water. After a second dusting with the powder the area should be left for 1 week at which time the procedure can be repeated if necessary. Five percent 5-fluorouracil cream is an alternative but more painful treatment. It is the best way of dealing with meatal warts of the penis. Lignocaine 5% ointment may be needed to relieve discomfort from treatment. Longstanding fibrous lesions will require cryotherapy, or diathermy under general anaesthetic; these treatments may be needed for pregnant women as the warts then grow more profusely due to increased vascularity. Podophyllin or 5% 5-fluorouracil should then not be used as they may damage the fetus and cause a peripheral neuropathy in the mother.

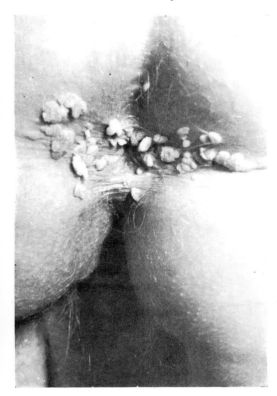

Fig. 55 Soft warts extending into the anal canal.

The destruction of warts can also be undertaken by freezing with carbon dioxide snow, as described on page 184. A painkiller or sedative should be given half an hour before the procedure begins and then any thick skin removed. Treatment is for between 30 seconds and 5 minutes, depending upon the size and depth of the lesion. A dressing is then required, having a circular pad to keep any pressure off the painful area. A week later the wart will be found in the roof of a blister, which can then be removed and the base painted with crystal violet 1% in spirit. Cryotherapy, as described on page 183, is a quicker treatment.

Dinitrochlorbenzene is a notorious sensitiser and can readily produce a local contact dermatitis. Applying it accurately until a reaction is produced has been advocated for the treatment of stubborn warts. The resulting skin changes hasten the development of immunity against the virus and thus the natural resolution of the lesion. However, when considering this and all the other sophisticated and potentially dangerous procedures, it is well to remember the natural history of the wart: 'Nature's cure is very acceptable because no trace of the wart is left, which is more than can be said for man's injudicious interference.' (Lyell).

Chapter 13. Infestations

Bites are reactions to chemicals, saliva or anticlotting agents that are injected so blood can be withdrawn by the insect. *Stings* are due to the poisonous venom that is injected either in defence or attack. The amount of reaction mainly depends on how allergic the patient is to the compound. For example, a bee-keeper who has become desensitised from previous stings may only develop an inflammatory papule, whereas a patient who is allergic may react violently and die. Systemic treatment, as for anaphylactic shock, may be needed. This would include injecting 1:1000 adrenaline subcutaneously (0.075 ml per minute up to a maximum of 1.0 ml), sodium hydrocortisone succinate 100 mg intravenously, and a quick-acting antihistamine intramuscularly. Sensitive patients should carry isoprenaline 10 mg or antihistamines to use sublingually. Fairly large doses of the last mentioned are needed. Very strong steroid alcoholic lotions, available for scalp treatment, should be applied to the lesions every few hours. The spirit base acts as an antiseptic which is an advantage, as not all horse flies 'scrub up' before operating!

Papular urticaria

Papular urticaria used to be called 'heat spots' or put down to a 'food allergy', but it is in fact due to an allergic reaction to multiple bites. The small, hard, irritating papules tend to group together in areas of tight clothing, or stretch out in a route depicting the animal's progress! The patient is actually allergic to the bites which can be from mites, fleas or lice. A bite then produces an itching urticarial area within half an hour, usually with a central punctum. A delayed hypersensitivity reaction may also develop at about 48 hours; this consists of persistent urticarial papules which last for several days and may flare up whenever the patient is rebitten elsewhere. Those who have become desensitised can be bitten with virtually nothing showing apart from an occasional central punctum. This is difficult to explain to an irate mother who has

135

brought one of her children covered in spots, some of which have become septic or have even blistered. Introduce the subject by saying that the child has become allergic to some biting mite which is common on all pets or birds. Don't use the word flea as it will evoke tremendous hostility even if they are of the non-human variety! Mother's co-operation is needed to track down the source of infestation. Sometimes this can be seen from the distribution of the rash, being more obvious on the forearms where pets are carried, or on the backs of legs from touching the sofa where the pet is allowed to sit. Real Sherlock Holmes work is sometimes needed, as fleas and mites may trek in from nests on the outside of a house when all the birds have flown!

The management of papular urticaria must include removing the source of infestation. Modern vacuum cleaners are effective on carpets and upholstered furniture. Pets must be disinfested even if they appear clear. Organophosphate preparations (Alugan) should be applied to cats as a powder and as a lotion to dogs. Benzene hexachloride powder, mentioned later, should be used on other pets. Local treatment for the lesions is with crotamiton (Eurax) hydrocortisone cream, though clioquinol together with an intermediate strength steroid is useful when there is secondary infection.

Pediculosis

Pediculosis is the infestation of the body surface by lice, and occurs under circumstances of poor personal hygiene. The louse is relatively harmless, usually producing only a slight host reaction. It is 3–4 mm in diameter, translucent, and oval in shape with no wings but six legs, each with a claw. It lives on fresh blood sucked from humans, and lays translucent eggs which develop into larvae after a week and into the adult louse 2 weeks later. There are 3 clinical types of pediculosis, each specific to the area of the body where it normally feeds.

Head lice

Pediculosis capitis is an infestation with head lice, and is more common in long and undisturbed hairstyles, or due to neglect. The louse fastens its eggs (nits) to the hair at skin level by means of a cylindrical sheath of chitin. As the hair grows they move away from the scalp. The presence of the nits is a characteristic finding, and occasionally the lice themselves may be seen. The infestation usually causes irritation and scratching may give rise to secondary infection in the form of an impetigo of the scalp. When this occurs there is commonly lymphadenopathy of the posterior cervical glands on the back of the neck.

Pubic lice

Pediculosis (phthirus) pubis is an infestation by pubic lice which usually follows venereal contact. It is the smallest louse of the group, being more rounded and crab-shaped, whereas the others are longer and thinner. The condition is important in the differential diagnosis of pruritus vulvae and ani but can also affect the eyelashes, chest and axillae. Itching is severe.

Body lice

Pediculosis corporis is an infestation by body lice, and has also been called 'vagabond's disease'. Unlike the head and pubic louse it lives in clothing except when feeding and lays white oval eggs in the seams. It is the largest pediculus and the resulting papules, excoriations and scabs may become pigmented if longstanding and neglected. Disinfestation of clothing is the important aspect of treatment, together with having a thorough bath.

Bedbugs

Bedbugs are still an important source of infestation in old buildings and old beds where they can survive for up to 2 months without feeding. They usually measure 3 × 4 mm, are oval, yellow-brown and have six legs. The bugs are attracted by the temperature of the host's skin; because of the warmth they can also be found in the backs of television sets! The bugs normally feed in darkness; the bites are therefore more common on the uncovered face and neck if the patient is bitten in bed. Eggs are laid in the crevices of skirting boards and furniture. Disinfestation should be carried out by the local health department, using preparations such as Fican W from Fisons. These require special precautions during application; accidental poisoning should be treated with atropine, the insecticide being an anticholinesterase.

Fleas

Fleas are brown and wingless but can jump several feet. Their eggs are laid between floorboards or in dust. The bites produce haemorrhagic spots, each surrounded by an itchy wheal and are mainly seen in groups, especially on trunk and limbs. Leaving on one's cycle clips, in certain houses in the village, was good advice from a predecessor on how to avoid being bitten!

Harvest mite

The harvest mite (harvester) is a similar cause of irritant and sensitivity reactions. Living mainly on low vegetation it needs certain proteins for its development. It attaches itself to the passing host and only drops off when its feed of digested skin is complete. The distribution of the lesions depends upon the type of clothing worn, occurring where the mite collects, typically just above the level of the belt and at the top of the socks. Infestations occur mainly in the late summer. The number of bites can be reduced by wearing clothing that covers the areas of contact with the mites; jeans and cycle clips are recommended! Afterwards the clothing should be changed and a bath or shower taken before the mites have had time to embed. Occasionally patients have to use insect repellents.

Food or grain mites also cause allergic reactions on areas of contact such as the flexor aspect of the forearms. Animal scabies can cause a similar papular eruption, which may resemble the human scabies except that burrows are not seen.

Scabies

Scabies is an infestation with the mite *Sarcoptes scabiei* (acarus), which is specific to humans. It has a relatively low degree of infectivity and is spread only by prolonged close contact plus poor personal hygiene, especially in bed and amongst children. It is just visible to the naked eye, the female being slightly less than 0.5 mm in diameter, and the male being half her size. It is a pearly grey colour and has eight legs.

The fertilised female burrows under the skin where she spends the rest of her life and lays up to 25 eggs. About 3 days later these hatch as six-legged larvae which move to the surface and shelter in the hair follicles. Here they develop into the full eight-legged adult after about 2 weeks. Mating then takes place and the fertilised female either starts a fresh burrow on the same host or during personal contact is transferred to infect another human.

After the incubation period of at least 1 month from the initial infestation, the host becomes sensitised to the presence of the mites or their debris. Severe itching occurs, especially when the patient is warm in bed at night. In adult patients the head and neck are never involved, probably due to the lower skin temperature. The rash has two components: a widespread papular eruption due to the wandering mites and burrows caused by the fertilised females. The burrows can be seen tracking intra-epidermally for up to 1 cm as an irregular greyish white line, with a darkened area at one end indicating the site of the female. They mainly occur in the clefts between fingers, on the flexor aspects of the wrists, on the palms, soles and around the ankles. Sensitisation at the site of the burrows causes scaling urticarial papules best visualised on the penis, breasts and anterior axillary folds. The allergic reaction is sometimes sufficient to cause a blister, but the burrow can often still be seen within its wall.

The diagnosis of scabies involves demonstrating the presence of the acarus. Often there is a history of pruritus in another member of the family or close friends. Once found, a burrow should be carefully opened at the closed end with a sewing needle parallel to the burrow (Fig. 56). The acarus usually sticks to the end of the needle and can then be transferred to a microscope slide. Caustic potash 10% solution applied to a burrow which is then scraped with a scalpel and transferred to the slide is a less effective method of visualising eggs or the acarus. Letting a patient who doubts the diagnosis look down the

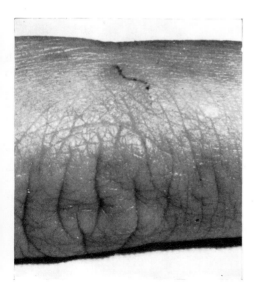

Fig. 56 Scabies showing characteristic burrow, with small dark bulge at the closed (nearest) end denoting site of female acarus.

microscope will certainly increase the chance of strict adherence to the instructions for treatment!

Secondary infection of the lesions is common, and it is occasionally necessary to use clioquinol with hydrocortisone cream for a couple of days before starting the stronger antiscabetic treatments to be described. Systemic antihistamines are useful when there is pruritus. Norwegian (crusted) scabies is due to widespread proliferation of the acari, due to the lack of scratching by the host. This usually occurs in mentally deficient patients and when systemic or local steroids have been used. Reinfection in a previously sensitised host will cause a pruritus within a few hours, which may succeed in dislodging the mite.

Treatment

Gamma benzene hexachloride

Gamma benzene hexachloride is the mainstay in the treatment of the pediculoses, fleas, bedbugs and scabies. It is available as a 1% cream (Lorexane) and a 1% lotion (Quellada). These preparations should be applied liberally after thorough cleaning and left in place for 24 hours before being washed off. Gamma benzene hexachloride is also available for the treatment of head lice as a 2% concentration in a detergent base (Lorexane No. 3) and a 1% concentration in a shampoo base (Quellada application). These should be applied to wet hair and well rubbed in for 4 minutes before rinsing. The following day these procedures should all be repeated for scabies and a week later for lice; a total change of clothing and bedding should accompany the last applications. Gamma benzene hexachloride is also available as a dusting powder for the disinfestation of pets and the areas where they sleep.

Dicophane

Dicophane is an alternative preparation, available as a 1% shampoo which also contains gamma benzene hexachloride 1% (Esoderm shampoo), for the treatment of head lice. It should be applied to the hair and left for 2–3 minutes before being rinsed out. The process should be repeated a week later. The same combination is available as a lotion which can be used in the treatment of scabies; it should be rubbed well in and allowed to dry. The procedure should be repeated on three successive nights, and on the third there should also be an accompanying total change of clothing and bedding, as detailed later under benzyl benzoate.

Malathion

Malathion is an alternative preparation for the treatment of resistant head and pubic lice. It is available as a 0.5% lotion (Prioderm lotion) which should be rubbed into the hair and left to dry. After 12 hours the hair should be shampooed and combed whilst wet. The whole procedure should be repeated after 1 week. Malathion is also available as a 1% shampoo (Prioderm shampoo) which should be well rubbed into wet hair and left for 5 minutes before being rinsed out and the application repeated. The whole procedure should be carried out again a week later. Malathion is irritant and inflammable, and therefore must not come into contact with the eyes or naked lights. After rinsing, hair can be combed just for aesthetic reasons to remove the dead nits.

Benzyl benzoate

Benzyl benzoate 25% application BP (also available as 25% emulsion, Ascabiol) is very effective for the treatment of scabies in adults. All close contacts must be treated, whether they appear affected or not, as they may be incubating the disease. After a thorough bath, all itchy spots and burrows should be scrubbed and the skin dried. The whole body surface, not just the affected areas, should then be painted with the benzyl benzoate from the chin downwards using a paintbrush. There must be special attention paid to the flexures and feet, and this is best carried out by a second person. The application should be allowed to dry, this being best effected by standing in a warm room. Unless this is thoroughly carried out by qualified staff, a second application should be made once the first has dried. The following evening a further thorough application is made, and then on the third evening there is a second bath to remove the benzyl benzoate; at the same time all personal linen and clothing should either be laundered or stored for 2 weeks in order to kill off any remaining acari. Any areas of skin that are washed during the 3 days of treatment should receive another application of the benzyl benzoate. Further use should be discouraged as the preparation is irritant.

Crotamiton

Crotamiton is available as a 10% lotion or cream (Eurax) and is the mainstay for the treatment of scabies in infants. It should be applied twice daily to the entire body, including the head and neck, until the eruption has improved. This usually takes about a week. After a bath, one thorough application of benzyl benzoate should then be made which should not be washed off for a further 48 hours.

Applications of crotamiton are also useful to relieve any persistent itching in adults after the benzyl benzoate treatment is completed. Failure to eradicate the infestation is due entirely to faulty technique or reinfection from an outside source:

> Even the vicar wrote in the parish magazine about the Itch. Children usually play together and come into intimate bodily contact, but it was to the adults that the magazine referred! The old family doctor was less bothered about the sanctity of marital life than the spread of scabies; as soon as he cured one family, someone living outside the flock would reintroduce it and the trouble would start all over again!
>
> During the wartime epidemic of scabies, it had been suggested that on a chosen day the entire nation should annoint themselves from the chin downwards with benzyl benzoate emulsion. Churchill rejected the advice as undemocratic!

Chapter 14. Leg ulcers

Gravitational ulcers

Whilst the majority of skin conditions are probably the result of civilisation, there are others which have been present since man adopted an upright posture. These are due to an increase in venous pressure in the lower limbs and are variously called 'gravitational', 'varicose', 'hypostatic' or 'hydrostatic' ulcers. They constitute nearly all of the leg ulcers and involve 0.5% of the British population.

Hippocrates was the first person to recognise an association between varicose veins and leg ulcers, but these varicosities do not normally cause any local change unless there is also valvular incompetence of the deep veins. There are some less common causes of ulceration, such as arteriosclerosis, whose treatment is different and therefore a correct diagnosis is necessary.

The arterial supply to the lower third of the leg is relatively poor, and hence any interference with the venous drainage of blood will greatly alter the perfusion and therefore viability of the tissues. The venous blood drains from the superficial blood vessels through the deep fascia and via the perforating veins to the deep femoral, which in turn drains into the vena cava. Valves throughout the system ensure one-way flow and this is especially important in the perforators. The number and location of the valves are a genetic variable; half the patients with varicose veins have a positive family history.

The pressure at any point in the veins depends upon the height of blood above it without the support of a competent valve. This is hydrostatic pressure and is therefore increased if the valves are damaged. The deep veins are supported by muscle and thick connective tissue and are therefore capable of withstanding pressure. Any further increase is unlikely to have any effect unless the valves in the perforating veins are damaged or become incompetent. In this case, the pressure is transmitted to the superficial veins which are unsupported, resulting in increasing dilation and viscosity. The increase will also cause the leakage of fluid into the tissues, which is known as oedema.

143

The return of venous blood mainly depends upon the muscle pump: during leg muscle contraction, blood is forced out of the leg and is prevented from flowing back by the valves. Virtually no pumping therefore takes place in a patient who sits still in a chair, or in those with the immobility of old age, arthritis or paralysis; reduced venous return also occurs from compression of the abdominal veins, as in pregnancy or tumours of the pelvis and in congestive heart failure. With reduced return there is stasis and more chance of venous thrombosis.

Thrombosis can occur when there is an increased coagulability of the blood. This is why deep-vein thrombosis may follow operations, pregnancy, and the taking of the contraceptive pill. Thrombosis may also follow trauma to the endothelium which is very easily damaged. The valves may be destroyed by a thrombosis, become incompetent due to thickening with age, or be congenitally absent or reduced in number. Recanalisation usually occurs following a deep-vein thrombosis, but the valves themselves do not repair. Incompetent valves increase the hydrostatic pressure on the area below, which causes oedema.

The onset of oedema is usually insidious, appearing first after long periods of standing and during the warmer weather. This is easily reversed by lying down, or by elevating the legs when in the seated position. If the oedema is allowed to persist, the condition may gradually progress through all the following stages, finally terminating in a gravitational ulcer and its complications:

Firstly a diffuse area of redness develops. This is followed by a progressive brown pigmentation due to the deposition of haemosiderin, from the destruction of red blood cells that have escaped from the capillaries. Minor trauma may then produce an ulcer with extending, irregular edges and an infected base. Less commonly ulceration follows the scratching of a previously existing area of gravitational eczema. Gravitational ulcers are not normally painful unless there is associated surrounding infection. Pseudomonas is then often the main organism involved. The pain produced causes immobility of the patient, which in turn will worsen the condition. Chronic infection may cause an anaemia which will further reduce the tissue viability.

Untreated, the gravitational ulcer not only makes the patient less independent (Fig. 57), but may also cause a psychological change. The ulcer arouses sympathy which accounts for much of the slow response to therapy! When this happens, there has usually been a failure to carry out the local treatment strictly and follow the general instructions, such as those given in the proforma at the end of this chapter.

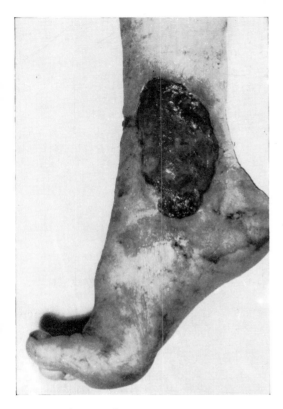

Fig. 57 Chronic gravitational ulcer with fixation of the ankle from previous lack of movement.

Arteriosclerotic ulcers

Arteriosclerotic ulcers must be differentiated from gravitational ulcers as compression will make them worse. Their treatment takes longer and they are particularly painful, being characteristically worse at night and with warmth. The ulcers affect older patients and usually occur below the ankles. They have a more punched-out appearance and are surrounded by erythema. On the other hand, gravitational ulcers tend to be present on either side of the leg, within 20 cm above the ankle. As the wearing of shoes acts as adequate support against gravitational changes, ulcers of the foot in the 'civilised' countries are usually due to arteriosclerosis (Fig. 58). The peripheral pulses may then be reduced or absent and calcification of the arteries felt, or seen on an X-ray of the soft tissues. Symptoms of intermittent claudication may also be present. Trauma and any constant pressure must be avoided, and foam dressings should be used. Compression bandages usually cause increased pain and worsen the condition. Superficial areas respond to

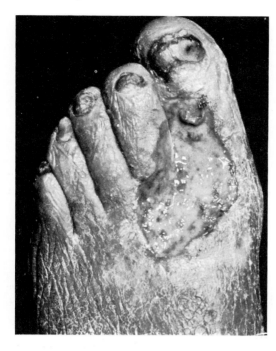

Fig. 58
Arteriosclerotic ulcer
with associated
atrophic scaling skin,
nail thickening, and the
absence of oedema.

dry dressings, powder and the occasional use of dyes. Deeper ulcers should be dressed with silver nitrate 0.5% chlorhexidine 0.2% cream.

Diabetic ulcers are usually due to arteriosclerotic changes. More rarely they are caused by the neuropathy, with diminished sensation in the limbs which are unknowingly traumatised. These ulcers are called trophic, are prone to infection and are abnormally slow to heal. They may also be caused by other rare neuropathies.

A number of other medical conditions either cause or aggravate leg ulcers. The important ones are hypertension, cardiac failure and anaemia; autoimmune disease such as rheumatoid arthritis occasionally causes ulceration. Infection by virulent pyogenic organisms, tertiary syphilis or tuberculosis occasionally causes ulceration. Specific systemic treatment is effective.

Chilblains may become ulcerated when severe. Unlike other leg ulcers they are more common in the young and usually itch. The extremities are effected by circumscribed oedematous erythematous areas. Chilblains are best prevented by exercise and by avoiding the cold. Central heating and the wearing of really warm clothing are the most important aspects of treatment. Patients in rented accommodation should be encouraged to purchase a suitable heater for use overnight.

The internal and external use of vasodilators such as nicotinic acid derivatives is of less importance but is sometimes helpful.

Management

The management of gravitational ulcers involves improving the venous return, treating any infection and dealing with any other underlying cause. The aim is also to prevent complications. Thrombosis and phlebitis are the most common, whereas cellulitis or haemorrhage occur less often.

Prophylaxis includes reducing the chance of thrombosis in susceptible patients who should avoid all unnecessary recumbency and be mobilised early, especially after operations. If a deep-vein thrombosis does occur, anticoagulants and firm bandaging will minimise any further extension or pulmonary emboli. Once valvular incompetence has occurred, venous support will be required *indefinitely* unless surgery or injection is carried out. It is obviously better to treat venous insufficiency at an early stage, before an ulcer develops. Elevating the feet, encouraging walking, avoiding standing, and the wearing of support stockings may be all that is required.

When sitting, the legs should always be elevated, the feet being higher than the hips. Those who are arthritic or overweight (or both) find this position uncomfortable at first, and require careful watching and encouragement; the patients have a tendency to lower their legs as soon as the nurse's back is turned. Patients must fully understand the aims of treatment, and to reinforce this should be given an instruction sheet similar to the proforma at the end of this chapter. Check that they know how to carry it out.

Bedrest is only needed when there is gross oedema, infection, ulceration or wet eczematisation. The foot of the bed should be elevated at least 23 cm, the sheets being kept off the legs by a cradle. Hospitalisation is necessary for the unteachable or uncooperative patient and for social reasons. Patients should be encouraged to get up for the toilet unless there are any overriding medical contraindications. This not only improves morale but also saves nursing time and reduces the development of complications.

Compression bandages should invariably be used for the treatment of gravitational leg ulcers. Their main function is to reduce oedema, and they therefore have to be applied when it is minimal before the patient gets out of bed. This can be done by the patients themselves once they have been taught exactly how. The bandages should be applied from the inside to the outside, starting over the toes and usually finishing at the mid-thighs. Cosmetically, flesh-coloured bandages are less noticeable.

Elasticated tubular stockinette (Tubigrip) gives the least support, but is the easiest to apply. Cotton elastic bandages (Elastoweb) give more support, whereas the one-way stretch bandages are even more effective but less popular because of their thickness. Elastic adhesive plaster (Elastoplast) is the most effective compression bandage. It should be reversed on those with hairy legs and then covered with talc and tubular gauze. It can then be left in place for up to a month. When there is eczematisation it should be applied over a zinc paste bandage in order to reduce the risk of sensitisation to the constituents of the plaster. The plaster and zinc paste combination is also useful for patients who would otherwise interfere with their dressings. A strip of the smallest tubular cotton gauze is a useful guide for the scissors when the dressings are removed. This strip should be left under the zinc paste avoiding the ulcer and the thick part of the dressings which occur anterior to the ankle. Deep ulcers benefit considerably from the use of pressure pads. These can be cut from foam-rubber and should conform to the shape and depth of the ulcer. They are then covered with the compression bandages.

Permanent support can be given by elastic stockings, which are more expensive. Unfortunately ointments and pastes spoil the elastic and the stockings are therefore reserved for patients who no longer require local treatment. The thicker ones give more support but are cosmetically less acceptable; medium weight two-way stretch with heels provide a good compromise. They should be measured to the mid-thighs for effectiveness and appearance. They need replacing at about 6-monthly intervals. Instructions on how patients can become used to wearing stockings are given in the proforma.

Physiotherapy is essential to increase mobility and improve circulation. Teaching of exercises is important, as patients can do so much to help themselves; they are essential for those who are bedridden. Ankle and leg movements, as detailed in the proforma, operate the muscle pump and improve circulation. The elderly have a tendency to curl up in bed with the development of contractures and pressure sores or even bronchopneumonia. Exercises and active physiotherapy are needed to prevent these occurring. The prevention and treatment of pressure sores are discussed in greater detail in Chapter 15. Physiotherapy is important to correct the lopsided, limping, shuffling gait that patients adopt to avoid the discomfort caused by the ulcer; this tends to reduce further the efficiency of the muscle pump and consequently worsens the condition. The range of physiotherapy includes encouraging walk-

ing with the compression bandage in place, heel-raising exercises to
prevent contractures, and massage to give physical assistance to venous
flow.

The lymphatics, like veins, also contain valves. The muscle pump
therefore maintains the flow of lymph up into the major lymphatics
and back into the general circulation. Upward massage of a limb has
the same effect and is the essence of the Bisgaard technique. This is even
more effective when the limb is elevated at 45°, as this also assists
drainage. Lymph contains protein which has considerable osmotic
pressure and must not therefore be allowed to collect in the tissues,
where it will attract further fluid.

Skin with gravitational changes is very delicate and prone to sensitisation; therefore nothing which is a known allergen should be used
in its treatment. Topical antibiotics should be avoided. Systemic antibiotics may be used if there is cellulitis; swabs will determine which
pathogens are present. Chlorhexidine, sodium hypochlorite solution
such as half-strength Milton, and the dyes are excellent for staphylococcal and streptococcal infections, while silver nitrate is very effective
against pseudomonas and proteus. More details are given in Fig. 76.
Most ulcers contain mixed infections. Alternating the treatments then
gives the best results but this should not be more frequently than once
a week as otherwise it will be impossible to monitor progress.

Epithelialisation can be delayed either by pathogenic organisms being
present in profusion or by the antiseptic being too strong; in this respect
silver nitrate 0.5% and chlorhexidine 0.2% in a cream or lotion is a very
good antiseptic combination which is not strong enough to delay
epithelialisation. Nurses should wear gloves when applying it in order to
prevent cross-infection or the silver staining their skin. When lotions
are used the gauze may stick to the newly formed epithelium; dressings
must therefore be moistened with further lotion before they are removed
(Fig. 59a–h).

Really dirty, infected ulcers are best cleaned by hydrogen peroxide
(10 vol.). This is applied liberally on cottonwool and left to effervesce.
It is then dabbed dry with gauze and the treatment repeated. Silver
nitrate with chlorhexidine 0.2% cream is then applied and left un-
touched for 24 hours. Occasional applications of crystal violet 0.5% in
water may be needed if staphylococcal infection persists.

Alternatively an infected ulcer can be cleaned with soaks of silver
nitrate 0.5% chlorhexidine 0.2% in water. Gauze swabs soaked in the
lotion are applied every 3 hours during the daytime and moistened twice
at night. This treatment requires adequate nursing staff and is only
suitable for in-patients. Failure to respond may be due to the presence

Fig. 59a–h   Dressing a
leg ulcer:

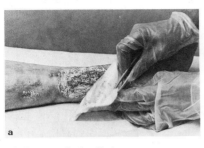

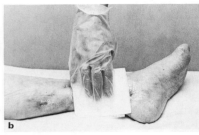

(a) Removal of soiled
gauze parallel to the
ulcer

(b) Gently drying with
clean gauze

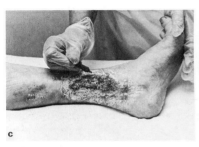

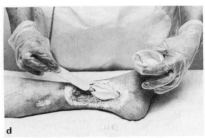

(c) Overgranulating
areas being treated by
rolling a silver nitrate
stick over them

(d) Application of
silver nitrate and
chlorhexidine cream
after applying
protective paste

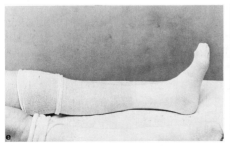

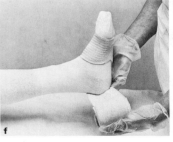

(e) The cream is finally
covered with gauze, a
light bandage and
tubular gauze

(f–h) Elastic web
bandage being applied
from the toes upwards

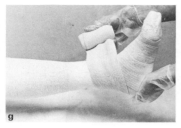
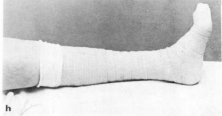

of anaerobic organisms. This is characterised by a layer of adherent, purulent, washleather slough. Metronidazole (Flagyl) should then be given systemically in addition to the local treatment.

Overgranulation delays epithelialisation and can be controlled by the careful use of a silver nitrate stick (usually 95%). After an analgesic has been given the stick should be rolled gently over the tissue until the surface colour changes to a milky grey.

Any sogginess or irritation of the skin surrounding the ulcer should be prevented by a protective application of phenoxyethanol 2% in zinc and salicylic acid paste BP (Fig. 59d). This should first be softened by creaming in the palm of the hand and then applied sparingly with the fingers right up to the edge of the ulcer. Cooking oil is useful for removing caked paste from the surrounding areas. The hands should be washed before and afterwards or gloves worn to prevent cross-infection. Moist varicose eczema can be quickly dried with clioquinol in an intermediate strength steroid cream; crystal violet 0.5% in calamine lotion BP is equally effective. A change can then be made to phenoxyethanol 2% in zinc and salicylic acid which is more protective. The secondary absorption eczema from varicose and contact dermatitis can usually be adequately treated with intermediate strength steroid creams, providing that the ulcer has been treated as already described.

Local treatment must be continued until the ulcerated areas have healed and are entirely smooth. Sometimes local scaling remains and this is easily traumatised, or picked off by the patient, causing fresh ulceration. Scales should therefore be treated with phenoxyethanol 2% in zinc and salicylic acid paste. Any resistant areas will respond to salicylic acid 5% ointment or urea 10% cream (Calmurid). Gross diffuse gravitational scaling is now very rare due to the increase in domiciliary nursing services (Plate 28). Treatment can be started with the salicylic acid 5% ointment and the strength gradually increased if required. When the hypertrophic keratin is soft it can be removed very carefully with a wooden spatula.

It is often useful to trace out the shape and size of the ulcer, so as to assess progress. The use of a thin polythene bag makes this simpler; first, a corner should be cut off for orientation, such as the top right. The ulcer is then traced gently with an easy flowing ballpoint pen and the soiled lower side of the bag cut off and discarded. This leaves a clean tracing for future reference.

If the tissue viability can be improved the body can do most of the healing on its own! Nature should be assisted with its own cure and therefore general medical care is important. Any underlying conditions such as cardiac failure, anaemia or diabetes will reduce the circulation and therefore tissue viability; these should be looked for and treated if found. Diuretics are required if there is oedema. Obesity should be avoided as it encourages immobility with failure of venous return. A balanced diet, however, is required, high in protein and vitamins, and including undercooked vegetables and salads for roughage to prevent constipation. Solid fats and carbohydrates should be reduced.

Surgery, in the form of pinch grafting, may be indicated when a chronic ulcer is clean and not infected. Details are given on page 186. It considerably reduces the healing time but is of no help if the arterial supply to the tissue is inadequate.

Fegan's injections involve treating the varicose and perforating veins with a sclerosing agent and following this up with exercises and compression bandaging for at least 6 weeks. Crockett's operation which involves saphenous vein ligation and stripping, together with tying off the perforators, may give excellent results.

Bandages provide a physical protection against damage to the friable tissue. The tissue will remain delicate for a long period after treatment, which is a further indication for indefinite bandaging. A watchful eye should be kept for neurotic excoriations as described on page 49, which may slow or even reverse any progress. Marking the bandages may be needed to discourage or to detect interference (Plate 29); elastic web cannot be marked effectively because of its stretchability, but the patient will find it impossible to reapply a marked cotton conforming bandage underneath it:

> She was the drudge of a large family with inadequate home accommodation. Her varicose veins developed after the birth of her last child 24 years ago. She was widowed 15 years later when she was 43. The ulcer followed a kick during a scuffle to get to the toilet. For the first time she had then been able to persuade her family to do things for her; but they made sure she attended out-patients and complained bitterly until she was admitted. In hospital the bandages were found to be frequently disturbed at nighttime. The skin surrounding the ulcer was excoriated, and the ulcer base was burnished as if it had been vigorously scrubbed with a rough towel. Progress was remarkably slow; the

burnished appearance persisted, despite the patient's protests that she never touched the ulcer as it was too sore. Later the consultant commented that more improvement had taken place in the last week than in the previous 7. The treatment had not been changed, so what had happened? It was the senior enrolled nurse who knew: the patient had confided that there was now something to live for—a 'nice gentleman' who had been visiting her had just proposed marriage!

If the causes are treated, trauma and standing are avoided, and elastic support is maintained indefinitely, then the prognosis for gravitational ulcers can be good. As with so many conditions, early treatment gives the best results.

Proforma: instructions to patients with gravitational eczema or ulceration

How can you help yourself?

The human body has been likened to an ingenious system of portable plumbing. Unfortunately, even the best systems break down; if you have a gravitational ulcer you will know how true this can be. In order to repair your particular system, it is essential first of all to assist the blood in your legs to return to your heart. Contrary to what most people think, the heart does not pump blood back to itself; this is done by the muscles in your legs during exercise, by squeezing the blood through the veins.

In order to get better you will almost certainly have to make some alterations to your established habits. Unpleasant as this may seem, the very fact remains that without your cooperation almost everything your doctor does to help you will fail to be of full benefit to you. If you want relief from your leg troubles, remember—it depends on you.

These are the things you can do to help yourself:

1 *Never stand still*

Plan your life so as to reduce to a minimum the time you spend standing still: Do you queue for cash desks in the shops, or for buses? Do you stand at counters, or in bars, or at parties? Do you stand talking to your friends? Do you stand watching football or other entertainments? Well, don't do it more than you can help! Remember, it isn't standing or just being on your feet that matters, it is the standing still which is harmful. When you have to be on your feet, shift from foot to foot; bend and straighten the knees a little from time to time; keep the toes moving inside your shoes. All these actions work the muscles of your legs and keep the blood moving. You will soon find that your legs stop aching and begin to feel more comfortable. What about work? Can you arrange either to do it sitting down for some of the time, or make some changes so that you keep moving while you are on your feet?

2   *Don't be afraid of exercise*

When you are wearing elastic bandages you should get as much exercise as possible, and should walk at least 2 or 3 miles each day. At the beginning of your treatment you may find this difficult, so you can do the following exercise instead: flexing your ankles up and down, either whilst standing or sitting, as if beating time to music. You should do this for at least 5 minutes every half hour.

3   *Avoid any obstructions to the veins*

Don't wear garters or any elastic around your legs. This is obvious; what is not so obvious is that constipation can cause harmful and unnecessary pressures on the veins. So don't allow yourself to get constipated. Senna (Senokot) is a safe laxative. Do not sit with your legs crossed. Never go to sleep in an armchair, such as watching television, or allow the edge of the seat to press into the backs of your legs, as this obstructs the veins.

4   *Assist the blood (from your legs) to return to your heart whilst resting*

The blood returns easily when your feet are higher than your heart. So when you rest don't just sit in a chair; put your feet up above the level of your hips. Take every opportunity you can during the day of resting with your feet up. The foot of your bed and couch must be raised at least 23 cm on wooden blocks, or 2 pairs of bricks wrapped in brown paper. You should never sit with the legs downwards or ever stand still except in exceptional circumstances.

5   *Keep your weight down*

Be warned in time; don't put on weight. Keeping your weight down is very much easier than having to reduce it on doctor's orders once you have allowed it to increase. Bread, buns, biscuits and pastries are the worst enemies, but there is nothing as fattening as food! Raw or undercooked vegetables are the least fattening, and also prevent constipation as they contain roughage.

6 *Bandage your legs correctly*

Best results are usually obtained by bandaging from the toe to the thigh. You will be shown how to put the bandages on, and make sure that you follow these instructions carefully. Do not allow the bandages to become slack or wrinkled, and replace them as soon as they lose their elasticity. Two types of bandage are mainly used:

a Elastic web (7.5 cm × 1.8 m). This is a cosmetically acceptable elastic bandage.

b Tubular shaped elastic bandage. This is rolled up on itself and then pulled on to the leg like a stocking.

If you apply your own bandages you should do so before getting out of bed. Do not bathe in the morning as this causes swelling of the legs. If your bandages feel tight after you have been wearing them for some hours, you should lie down with your legs elevated on the arms of a couch for an hour. Consult your own doctor if this does not bring relief. Wear lace-up shoes. If you feel hot and tired at the end of the day, change into another pair of lace-up shoes but not slippers.

7 *Do not let your legs get cold*

People with bad circulation usually make a deliberate effort to keep their hands warm, as cold ones are uncomfortable. Your legs are far less sensitive; they often get cold without your realising it, though you can tell quickly enough if you put your hand on your kneecap. Keep your legs warm but do not sit close to the fire.

As soon as the areas heal, then medium weight two-way stretch elastic stockings with heels, measured to the mid-thighs, may be prescribed for you. At first the stockings should be worn for a short time each day until the skin of your legs grows accustomed to them, and whilst this is happening you should wear your elastic bandages for all the rest of the day. Talcum powder should be applied to the legs for a while to make the stockings feel more comfortable. Remember it is no good leaving them off on occasions when you think you will look smarter without them. Medium- or light-weight stockings can be worn just for special occasions. Close attention to detail guarantees healing.

Chapter 15. Some problems in the elderly

Purpura in old age

Old age comes to some faster than others. Sometimes it is the mind that alters first, sometimes the skin. Exposure to sunlight over the years causes degeneration of the dermal collagen, making the skin look old and wrinkled (Fig. 66). Purpura is common from minor injury as the collagen no longer supports the blood vessels. Even helping a patient to walk by holding their forearm may produce a purpuric area which can alarm an anxious relative. These areas have a characteristic reticulate appearance with a clear-cut margin and take about a fortnight to clear. Scarring is sometimes produced. It is unfortunate that they are called senile purpura as often the patients are anything but senile:

She came into out-patients at the skin clinic with a Mona Lisa smile and a chain of scars down the right side of her neck. She looked all of 70 years old, with the hint of an ageless charm and two wedding rings on her finger. Seemed to have come to play some guessing game with the consultant, registrar, houseman, and anyone else to pay court. The note from her doctor asked what the marks were, and what to do about them. They had started soon after she had married her second husband, a couple of years ago now. She smiled with a challenging silence. The consultant's face reflected an urgent hotline conference with the Deity to pronounce some *ex cathedra* diagnosis—no reply. The registrar's more modern computer brain retrieved a morsel of his omnivorous taste for the more exotic literature, with an unconvincing print-out—pseudocicatrix de Colomb. No one seemed to be sure what it was. The houseman kept tactfully silent.

There were the scars winking back. A dozen small stellate lesions, about 20 mm in diameter, all down her right sternomastoid, the highest peeping coyly from behind her right ear and the lowest somewhere around the costosternal junction of her third rib. Most of the upper ones showed white scar tissue, like senile purpura sometimes leaves its trace, but nothing similar to be seen elsewhere on her body. The houseman remarked that the lower ones looked pinkly more recent as some purpura was still present.

Something stirred deep in the consultant's mind—memories of a stay in Paris long ago, when gallant men kissed married ladies' hands to whet the appetites of love; memories of starting lightly on the perfumed dorsum of a hand, bridging the wrist, nibbling up the forearm, nuzzling deeper into the dermis over the deltoid, and all-consuming passion past the clavicle. Madame still bears with elegance the jewellery of stellate scars on one arm, along with other souvenirs of springtime at Auteuil and a villa in Sologne.

Whether or not our old lady's partner also had star-shaped crowns on his dentures is perhaps more within the province of forensic medicine than dermatology, but at least not all of his weapons are too blunt to use. Our spinster lady typist looks modestly abashed at the case sheet diagnosis—geriatric love bites.

A sense of humour is a great asset and helps to keep perspective as nursing the elderly requires much time, patience and tolerance. Treatment must be with confidence but never arrogance. Be persistent, especially when attempting to mobilise them, but allow them to preserve their dignity. Above all, show them that you really care.

Skin changes

The skin undergoes typical changes with age. A decrease in sebum production results in cracking and in some cases asteatotic eczema. There is also a decreased resistance to chemical irritants. Bathing should be reduced and emulsifying ointment used instead of soap, as in the treatment of senile pruritis, discussed on page 103. Apart from senile purpura just described, exposed areas show an increased incidence of telangiectasia, keratoses, lentigines, leukoplakia, basal-cell carcinomas, and squamous-cell carcinomas.

Self-neglect

There is a tendency to self-neglect, not only due to cerebral arteriosclerotic changes, but also due to the increased physical difficulty in carrying out quite simple actions; if left uncut the toenails become thickened and curl back upon themselves (onychogryphosis), becoming very painful and damaging the skin. Infection may then take hold in the presence of poor tissue viability and lack of hygiene.

Malnutrition

Food preparation also becomes more difficult and the diet becomes inadequate with resulting poor health. Malnutrition is more common amongst those who live alone or who have gastrointestinal disease, especially when there is malabsorption. The loss of nutrients through neglected chronic ulcers or widespread skin rashes can further worsen the patient's general condition. The aim in management is to correct any underlying medical problem or deficiency and to encourage an active life with improved general health.

The bedridden elderly

Once bedridden, the elderly patient is very susceptible to several medical complications. Inactivity of the venous muscle pump in the legs results in an increased incidence of deep-vein thrombosis and consequent pulmonary emboli. Poor ventilation of the lungs also leads to an increased incidence of chest infections, especially in the debilitated.

Pressure sores

Pressure sores will occur if the patient is allowed to remain in one position for any length of time. They are due to the body weight causing compression of blood vessels and tissues over the bony prominences with resulting ischaemia and ulceration. The skin passes through the stages of a temporary then persistent erythema, blister formation, and finally an ulcer develops with sloughing and infection. Common sites include the sacral and ischeal areas of the back and the heels (Plate 30). If the patients are lying on their sides the femoral trochanter, knee, or lateral malleolus may be involved. The sores can develop within a matter of hours and prevention is very important as they usually take weeks or months to heal. They can occur in a healthy but unconscious adult though are more common in the elderly when there are circulatory problems and immobility. Oversedation can cause immobility and it should not be forgotten that older persons are often more affected by hypnotics or tranquillisers than are the young.

During normal sleep there is adequate movement of the body position to prevent any localised pressure changes. Severe pain, such as is experienced with arthritis, can cause a conscious reduction in movement with ensuing changes. The medical conditions discussed in Chapter 14 can cause a decrease in the viability of the skin making it easily damaged.

With correct nursing and management, pressure sores should not occur.

Management

Susceptible patients must wherever possible have urgent treatment of any underlying condition. They should be turned from side to side every 2 hours and use made of foam rubber rings to spread the body weight. Sheepskins or pads filled with polystyrene micronodules are also very effective. Padded rings should be made to keep weight off the heels. Painful red areas on the feet should always be protected. Macarthy's medical sheepskin bootees are helpful for the treatment of pressure sores of the heels, as they distribute the weight and give protection. Alternatively, bootees made from absorbent non-adherent foam dressing can be used, covered with tubular gauze. If available, water or ripple beds, or hammocks may obviate the need for these procedures. Patients should sit out of bed in a comfortable padded chair for as long as possible each day provided their position is changed from time to time. Care should be taken when moving a passive patient to lift him clear of the sheets; this is to prevent the trauma from any shearing action on the skin when being dragged on the bed.

The sheets should be clean, dry and not wrinkled, in order to prevent localised pressure. The skin should also be kept clean and dry, using soap and a soft sponge, drying by patting with a soft towel, never rubbing. Talc absorbs sweat and reduces friction. This can be supplemented by a lotion with an alcohol base if sweating tends to be excessive.

Incontinence may be a problem in the aged. The fundamental way of treating this is by retraining, but this is very time-consuming. The skin should be protected by a silicone barrier cream, zinc and castor oil or oily cream BP. Keeping the patient clean and dry by frequently changing the clothing prevents the development of a macerated and secondarily infected dermatitis, which in turn may be followed by sores in pressure areas. Benzalkonium chloride with cetrimide cream, clioquinol cream or even crystal violet 0.5% in calamine lotion may then have to be used. Undue sweating may also cause maceration and should be avoided by separating the limbs, the use of a cradle and keeping the patient cooler.

A high calorie and protein diet becomes even more essential once a pressure sore has developed. Locally, daily irrigation with saline and hydrogen peroxide helps to wash out pus and debris and discourages the anaerobic pathogens. A cream such as silver nitrate 0.5% with chlorhexidine 0.2% can then be applied. For a sore that is deep, soak the gauze in the cream before packing. The skin flora should be monitored by regular swabs for culture. Ultraviolet light may help keep down local infection and promote healing. Systemic antibiotics may be required if there is any cellulitis or systemic spread. Skin grafting may be required to aid the healing of extensive ulcers.

Infection in the elderly

Infection is more difficult to control in diabetics and the diagnosis should always be considered in resistant cases. There is an increased incidence of cellulitis, intertrigo, boils, carbuncles, pruritus vulvae and ani, and balanitis, the management of which have already been dealt with. There is an acceleration of the normal arteriosclerotic vascular changes in elderly patients who are diabetics; this can cause ischaemia, necrosis and ulceration at the peripheral ends of the limbs.

Infection in the elderly must be prevented especially if they are diabetics, meticulous care being taken of all cuts. Swabs and scrapings should be taken to see if pathogenic bacteria and fungi are present as detailed from page 190. The appropriate antibacterial or fungicidal powders or creams can then be applied. Systemic medications are usually only required if there is a systemic spread of infection. Rest, warmth provided it does not cause sweating, and observation of progress is required. Sedation, usually with antihistamines, is useful to prevent scratching, especially at night. Great care is required in the management of bunions, corns and overgrown toe nails, as mentioned in the section on chiropody on page 197. Shoes should be well-padded on the inside and never a tight fit.

Disease in old age

All in-patients, and especially the elderly, should be encouraged to get out of bed for the toilet unless there is a definite medical contraindication. This helps prevent pressure sores and other complications and also tends to keep the patient mobile and independent; it retains their dignity. Periods of admission should be kept to a minimum in order to prevent the elderly from becoming institutionalised; after 1 month it is better to discharge the patient whenever possible, even if this means readmission at a later date. After an unavoidably prolonged hospital stay, patients should be allowed home for a few days at a time, while they regain confidence that they can manage again on their own.

Following an illness, nurses, doctors, social workers and physiotherapists are all involved in rehabilitation. The family that is caring for the patient will need reassurance, advice and support. The community nurse may visit regularly and build up a good relationship, ensuring a quick medical and social response in a crisis. The social worker and health visitor can arrange 'meals-on-wheels', chiropody, walking aids, laundry services and home-helps as required. The family doctor will coordinate these services while undertaking the medical treatment. This not only 'saves' a hospital bed but can prevent a patient becoming institutionalised with loss of the will to live.

Age is not a disease; it is a part of life which must be accepted as ever changing. It is important that the elderly are not expected to conform to a pattern of dependency with avoidance of activity and fear of adversity; they should be allowed to fulfil to the end their potential to be themselves.

Rashes in the elderly have similar causes to those in young people, although the upsets sometimes appear more minor; even a small fall on the pavement can destroy confidence and be the start of complete withdrawal from life. Fear of death may be suppressed, but the old are frequently reminded of it as friends and relatives in their own age group die. Loneliness is an unhappy state:

> He was certainly a young-looking 87. His longstanding eczema developed
> 2 days after seeing his wife run over and killed outside his house. 'It was
> a terrible thing to see. I still get nightmares about it even though it was
> 15 years ago. I've been on my own since then. Nothing takes the place
> of someone with whom you have really shared your life.'

Chapter 16. Tumours—benign and malignant

A tumour is an abnormal mass of cells. Benign tumours remain localised and are much more numerous than the malignant variety.

Benign tumours

Many are congenital but some are noticed later in life, even though the cells forming them were present at birth. When the cells are derived from embryonic tissue they are called naevi or hamartomas. They have been classified histologically into many varieties depending on the predominant type of cell. Reference books should be consulted if these details are needed.

The mole

The mole is the commonest benign tumour. There are several on each person. Moles can be classified more simply on a therapeutic basis into pigmented or fleshy. Melanocytes are the cause of pigmentation; when this is obvious the lesion should either be left alone or totally excised because partial excision or repeated trauma may, in time, be followed by the development of malignancy. Pigmented moles on the soles and other areas where there is chronic irritation should therefore be excised. The lesions virtually never become malignant before puberty, so treatment can be left until the child is not only cooperative but actually wishes to have the blemish removed. This is important from the psychological point of view.

Old wives' tales are sometimes based on clinical observations! One is that it is dangerous to excise a pigmented lesion. While this is incorrect it is easy to see how the belief has arisen. The patient's attention is drawn to a pigmented mole because of increasing size, change in colour, friability, bleeding or irritation. These may be signs of malignancy. The patient then seeks attention but already it may be too late. Always excise a pigmented lesion that is enlarging so that the diagnosis can be checked by histology. Infection is the commonest cause but it is much more prudent to be certain. The chance of malignant change taking place within a year in pigmented naevi is about one in a million. Surgery should be avoided wherever possible as the resultant scars may be more unsightly than the original lesion.

Large pigmented hairy naevi may develop malignancy later in life. They are the province of the plastic surgeon who frequently has to treat them in stages because of their size. This should be completed before puberty as the development of malignancy is extremely rare before this time.

The fleshy mole is so amenable to dermatological treatment that it is given its own paragraph! Cautery, as will be described on page 180, can remove it without leaving a scar.

Seborrhoeic keratoses

Seborrhoeic keratoses are also called basal-celled papillomas or seborrhoeic warts. They are late-appearing naevi from about 40 years onwards, and increase with age. They usually occur on areas of skin normally covered by clothing and are seen more frequently in the 'white' races. They are not true warts as they are not viral in origin and are not usually associated with seborrhoea. There may be a dominant genetic tendency. The lesions give the appearance of being stuck to the skin, being round or oval, slightly raised papules up to 2 cm in diameter, which may be greasy in the early stages. Initially they are yellow-brown, becoming darker as they enlarge, with a rough raised surface. They have to be differentiated from pigmented naevi which are noticed at or soon after birth and tend to be smoother.

Treatment is only necessary for cosmetic reasons. The softer lesions usually respond within a month to precipitated sulphur 3% in a salicylic acid 3% ointment. Initially this should be applied sparingly and accurately at night-time but as tolerance is achieved, the treatment can be twice daily. The sulphur occasionally produces a branny scaling reaction of the surrounding skin. This quickly clears if treatment is temporarily suspended. The strength of both ingredients in the ointment can be doubled a few weeks later if resolution is not taking place. Alternatively quicker destructive treatment can be carried out either by cryotherapy, trichloracetic acid or cautery, as described from page 180.

Skin tags are seborrhoeic keratoses in which the connective tissue component is predominant. Treatment is given on page 185.

Haemangiomas

Haemangiomas are vascular naevi, which are congenital, benign tumours composed of capillaries. They are usually present at birth or shortly afterwards. All blanch on pressure.

A strawberry mark is a simple vascular naevus which mimics a strawberry, being raised, bright red and usually single. They are composed of a proliferation and dilation of capillaries forming cavernous spaces. The majority resolve spontaneously after the age of 5, though growth takes place for up to the first year and a half. Mothers need reassurance that provided they are patient, nature will heal the lesion far more perfectly than by destructive methods. They should also be told that any bleeding that may occur from trauma will be minimal and easily stopped by steady pressure with the aid of a clean handkerchief or tissue. Only rarely will plastic surgery be needed at about the age of 8 to tidy up a little loose skin. Very rarely the lesion is grotesquely large and may interfere with the development of binocular vision; a short course of oral prednisolone is then justified.

The *port wine stain* is a flat vascular lesion due to dilation of mature capillaries, also known as naevus flammeus (Fig. 60). The macular, diffuse telangiectasia has an irregular outline, usually unilateral, and is commonly seen on the face and the neck. Unfortunately it may also involve underlying structures. Epilepsy can occur if the brain is involved, and calcification is then seen on X-ray of the skull. A widespread naevus flammeus of the limb may be associated with increase growth due to excess vascularity at the epiphyses. Unlike the strawberry mark, naevus flammeus does not resolve, with one exception—a superficial triangular pale lesion in the centre of a baby's forehead, which disappears within a year of birth.

Treatment of haemangiomas. Cosmetic creams are the best treatment for unsightly lesions, especially after they have been paled by Grenz rays, described on page 195. Surgical intervention usually gives unsatisfactory results, though dermabrasion may produce a fine scarring that is more easily camouflaged.

Covering creams are often the best answer to unsightly problems, particularly in women who in any case may be using cosmetics. The creams are special formulations designed to give a good masking effect. Obtaining the correct shade is important and help may be sought from experts in large perfumery stores. Only allow purchase of the five basic

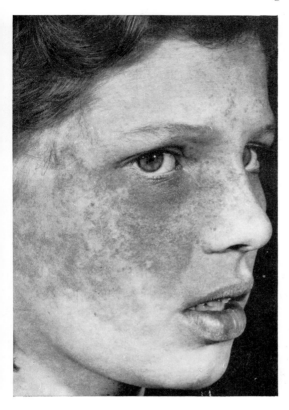

Fig. 60 Naevus flammeus.

essentials, otherwise much money will be wasted! These are masking cream, talcum, normal face powder, normal liquid make-up and cold cream.

After washing the skin with soap and water, dry carefully and apply the masking cream in small quantities with the ball of the finger, methodically working from the centre of the disfigurement with a tapping motion until the whole area is covered. At the junction of the blemish with normal skin feather the cream out with light strokes until the edge is disguised. Next press the talcum powder on using cotton-wool until the whole area is covered. After leaving to set for 10 minutes, use slightly damp cottonwool or a cosmetic brush to remove surplus powder. This should be done in the same direction of any small down-hairs to keep the powder and cream smooth. The normal liquid make-up should then be applied and care taken to smooth it lightly over the disguised area. Follow with normal face powder if desired. Before going to bed all make-up should be removed with cold cream and the area then washed with soap and water to clear any remaining grease. Covering creams from Elizabeth Arden, Boots, Innoxa and Medexport can usually be obtained on the National Health Service for the treatment of disfigurements.

Spider naevi

Spider naevi are acquired vascular naevi. They are composed of a central arteriole surrounded by radiating capillaries. These tend to appear spontaneously in childhood and pregnancy, liver or bleeding disorders. Cosmetic treatment is by diathermy or cautery to the central arteriole, as described on page 181.

Cherry angiomas

Cherry angiomas, known also as Campbell de Morgan spots, are seen in adults. They appear within a week of increases in temperature. The smallest may be misdiagnosed as petechiae unless a lens is used, their vascular nature then being obvious. Those smaller than 1 mm tend to disappear within a fortnight but the larger ones remain. Histologically they consist of collections of capillaries, some dilated, in the upper dermis. Treatment is unnecessary except for cosmetic reasons and can then be carried out with the cryoprobe jet, as described on page 183.

Keloids

A keloid is an excessive scar and is an acquired condition in that it usually follows trauma (Fig. 61). However, there is also a racial as well as a genetic tendency and certain sites such as the sternum are more prone to the disorder than others. There is a gradual development of a smooth, ridged tumour following the shape of the trauma, of which burns are the most common. The colour is pink initially, gradually fading to white with ageing. Early lesions may respond to the application of strong steroids. These are best given intralesionally, either by a pressure jet (Dermojet) or by injection. 4–6 treatments at weekly intervals are usually effective. In addition very strong steroids can be applied accurately daily, either as a tape or ointment and localised with adhesive strapping. Alternatively treatment can be with cryotherapy. Longstanding lesions may need excising but the patients should be warned of recurrence. X- or Grenz rays, described on page 194 and given both before and after surgery, seem to prevent this happening.

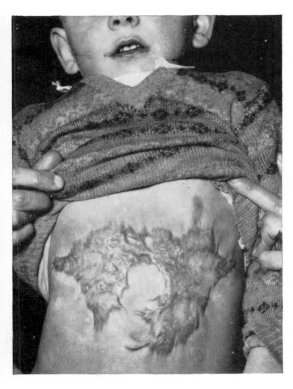

Fig. 61 Keloid following a scald.

Pyogenic granulomas

A pyogenic granuloma is a benign acquired lesion believed to follow a minor penetrating injury and commonly affects the fingers and scalp. There is a rapid proliferation of new capillaries which become dilated into a soft bright red 'raspberry-like' nodule up to 1.5 cm in diameter, with a smooth but sometimes ulcerated surface which occasionally bleeds easily (Plate 31). Treatment is by curettage under local anaesthesia followed by cauterisation or cryotherapy, as described on pages 180 and 183 respectively.

Chondrodermatitis helicis

Chondrodermatitis helicis is a benign acquired condition where there is chronic inflammation of the circumference of the external ear. It is due to chronic exposure to sunlight, cold and recurrent trauma. Males are more often affected than females, the sudden degeneration of the cartilage causing a very tender, hard, reddish nodule, often with an overlying crust. Patients are unable to sleep on the affected side. The extreme tenderness tends to distinguish this lesion from solar keratosis, but a squamous-cell carcinoma can sometimes be painful. Treatment is by surgical excision of the cartilage and overlying skin.

Dermatofibroma

Dermatofibroma, also known as histiocytoma, is a benign tumour of the fibrous component in the skin. These present as firm, shiny, painless well-defined nodules, and are probably a fibrous reaction to bites. They are more numerous on the limbs than the trunk and are harmless, only requiring excision for cosmetic reasons.

Lipomas

Lipomas are benign acquired tumours composed of dermal fat cells which proliferate into compressible 'domes', are single or multiple, and usually occur on the back, shoulders or scalp. Unless a rapid growth or change of nature is observed, excision is only recommended for cosmetic reasons.

Lentigo

Lentigo is a benign condition in which an increased number of melanocytes cause circular brown macules, darker than freckles and which do not darken in the sun. They appear in childhood, pregnancy and Addison's disease, but are usually just a cosmetic problem. The appropriate use of make-up is recommended, but they can be treated with cryotherapy if desired.

Neurofibromata

Neurofibromata are benign tumours composed of the fibrous tissue originating from the nerve sheaths. They can be felt as a hard nodule on the route of a major nerve. Superficial neurofibromas are up to 1 cm in diameter and commonly appear in pregnancy. Multiple superficial neurofibromatosis (Von Recklinghausen's disease) is a syndrome in which the widespread and often large, pedunculated, flabby flesh or brown tumours are associated with brown macules. The latter, 'cafe-au-lait' areas, may occur on their own.

Malignant change in multiple neurofibromatosis is very rare but the numerous lesions need observation at regular intervals. Excision is required for lesions that are enlarging and also for cosmetic reasons.

Adenoma sebaceum

Adenoma sebaceum is an inherited disorder consisting of small multiple flesh and pink papules on the face but especially the nasolabial folds. Periungual fibromata are often present as well as flat fibromatous naevi on the skin. Cafe-au-lait patches may also be seen. The earliest lesion to develop in infancy is a pale area like an ash tree leaf, most easily seen under the Wood's light. Lesions may affect other organs such as the brain when the condition is called tuberose sclerosis, and epiloia when there is epilepsy; mental retardation may then be present. There is a slight genetic overlap between this condition and multiple neurofibromatosis. Cosmetic treatment of facial lesions is by crotherapy, cautery under general anaesthesia or dermabrasion, depending on their extent.

Kerato-acanthoma

Kerato-acanthoma (molluscum sebaceum) are benign tumours but with histological features similar to squamous-cell carcinoma. They are more common following excessive exposure to sunlight on the face and men are more often affected. There is a very rapid initial growth, up to 5 cm diameter, of a flesh coloured dome-shaped lesion, which has a central crater (Fig. 62) containing a plug of keratin. The sides of the crater usually show telangiectasia. The lesions grow for a few weeks and spontaneously resolve over the following 3–6 months, leaving a cratered scar. Some tissue should be taken for histological examination to exclude squamous-cell carcinoma. What remains of the lesion should then be treated to reduce scarring either by half a cancer-treatment dose of X-rays or by curettage and cauterisation.

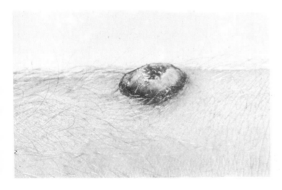

Fig. 62 Kerato-acanthoma showing a dome-shaped lesion with cratered centre.

Solar keratosis

Solar keratosis is an acquired premalignant condition due to chronic exposure to ultraviolet light. The skin overgrows as if to protect itself and forms multiple horny papules with dry adherent scales (Plate 32). It is more common in fair-skinned individuals who have less protective pigment and occurs after 40 years of age but usually between 65 and 75. It is necessary to watch the lesions carefully. If there is enlargement or a surrounding inflammation, biopsy should be carried out as carcinomatous change may then be taking place. Treatment if required consists of either cryotherapy or 5-fluorouracil 5% cream for 3–4 weeks, as described on page 183.

Leukoplakia

Leukoplakia is another premalignant condition, but while still benign (leukokeratosis) the cells are overgrowing and malignant change may ultimately develop. It is believed to be caused by chronic irritation. In the mouth this may be due to smoking or the presence of jagged teeth. It can also be caused by chronic infection such as syphilis. Patients complain of sensitivity to spicy or hot food. The mucous membranes usually of the mouth (but also of the vulva) develop a hyperkeratosis, which appears as a white well-defined thickening. Any irritants must be removed and dental attention arranged. Smoking is forbidden. If the condition has not resolved within 2 months biopsy should be undertaken to exclude the development of squamous-cell carcinoma. Cryotherapy is effective in the premalignant stage.

Malignant tumours

Malignant tumours are due to masses of abnormal cells dividing rapidly at the expense of the body into which they are spreading. The spread causes secondary metastases elsewhere and is either by direct extension or via the blood vessels and lymphatics. The composition of the tumour depends upon the type of cell from which the lesion originated. The degree of malignancy varies from tumour to tumour; in the more malignant the cells are less recognisable, more bizarre histologically and have a greater tendency to metastasise.

Any substance which tends to produce malignant change in a benign tumour or in apparently normal tissue is called a carcinogen; prolonged contact with the cells and adequate concentrations are usually needed. Tars and oils are examples of carcinogens, as is radiation from natural or man-made sources such as X-rays.

Tumours of the skin have the advantage of being visible and are therefore easily noticed by the patient at an early stage. They are then accessible for examination and diagnosis, which nearly always results in an improved prognosis.

Paget's disease

Paget's disease of the nipple is a rare skin change associated with an underlying malignancy within the breast tissue. The carcinoma grows back along the ducts and then spreads within the epidermis of the skin. It commonly affects females in the 40–60 age group, appearing as a unilateral eczema, progressing to infiltration, induration and nipple retraction. Later there may be ulceration and metastases. Treatment should be early by surgery, with or without X-ray therapy.

Intra-epidermal carcinoma

Intra-epidermal carcinoma is a localised squamous-cell malignancy where all the growth takes place initially in the epidermis. It is also called Bowen's disease. The area looks like infiltrated but localised unilateral patches of eczema, as does Paget's disease. After confirmatory biopsy they are best treated by cryotherapy. Once the cells are not contained by the epidermis they form a skin malignancy, exactly the same as the following to be described.

Squamous-cell carcinoma

Squamous-cell carcinoma commonly metastasise unless treated early. The lesions occur in the elderly, usually in areas subjected to chronic irritation and infection, trauma, chemicals such as light or shale oils, and in areas of leukoplakia, solar keratosis and arsenical keratosis. They develop as hard warty overgrowths which gradually enlarge to 1–2 cm diameter, when they usually ulcerate, leaving typical everted edges (Fig. 63). Treatment is by excision or radiotherapy.

Basal-cell carcinoma

Basal-cell carcinoma is a common tumour and constitutes 70% of all malignant skin tumours. It is also known as rodent ulcer or basal-cell epithelioma. The lesions are slow-growing and only locally invasive; infiltration of bone is rare but relentless (Plate 33). Basal-cell carcinomas commonly affect males over 40 years of age and especially appear

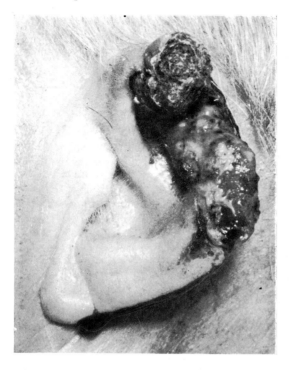

Fig. 63 Squamous-cell carcinoma showing ulceration and everted edges.

to occur in solar damaged skin, or are noticed following minor trauma to the face, forehead and scalp. There is an insidious onset of a nodule often with a pearly, waxy, raised edge, showing telangectasia. The lesions usually bleed and ulceration is common (Fig. 64). Basal-cell carcinoma should be suspected in any case of a sore that does not heal. Scraping it is usually not painful, and often reveals typical gelatinous material. The diagnosis can be confirmed either by cytology or biopsy; treatment is by cryotherapy, or plastic surgery for middle-aged patients and radiotherapy for the aged.

Malignant melanoma

Malignant melanoma is fortunately the rarest primary skin tumour but on the other hand is the most malignant and accounts for half the deaths from skin tumours. It metastasises very early and may present purely as the secondary growths even before the primary is noticed. The majority arise in pigmented naevi or on skin that has been damaged or irritated by sunshine and trauma over many years. It usually appears

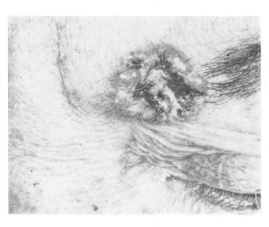

Fig. 64 Basal-cell carcinoma showing telangiectatic and nodular waxy edge surrounding areas of ulceration.

as a jet black nodule (Fig. 65a, b), sometimes with a red surround due to host immunity. Occasionally it lacks pigment perhaps due to rapid growth, and is then called amelanotic. Treatment is by urgent wide and deep excision, followed by removal of the lymphatic glands which drain the area if they are enlarged.

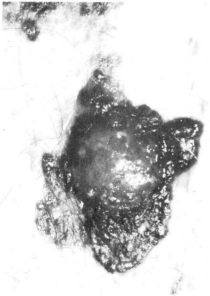

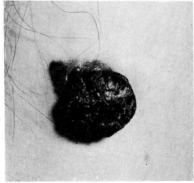

Fig. 65a & b
Malignant melanoma presenting as a jet black nodule (a) and with satellite metastases (b).

Malignant lentigo

Malignant lentigo is an intra-epidermal malignant melanoma. It occurs in the aged as a dark, slowly spreading 'senile freckle', usually on an exposed area such as the face (Fig. 66). After confirmatory biopsy the area can either be totally excised and grafted, or treated by cryotherapy and carefully followed up. The prognosis is good provided the malignant cells have been contained within the epidermis; otherwise it is similar to that of malignant melanoma just described.

Mycosis fungoides

Mycosis fungoides despite its name is not an infection but a very rare and invariably fatal malignant primary tumour, a reticulosis arising in the skin. Adult males are more often affected and without treatment death may occur within 5 years. The lesion starts as a non-specific pruritic rash, often misdiagnosed as eczema or psoriasis, and may last for months or even years. The areas extend and slowly become telangiectatic and infiltrated (Fig. 67). Mushroom-like tumours arise from these areas and ultimately ulcerate (Fig. 68). PUVA therapy described

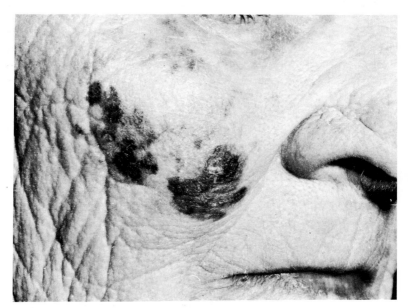

Fig. 66 Malignant lentigo showing as dark superficial tumours on a cheek with numerous wrinkles from sun exposure over many years.

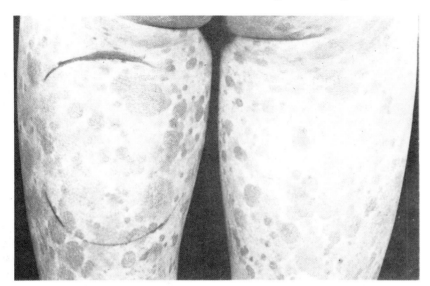

Fig. 67 Mycosis fungoides showing early infiltrated lesions.

on page 192 is probably the best initial treatment. Grenz rays are also effective and keep the condition quiescent for long periods. Their action can be potentiated by psoralens as in PUVA treatment. More resistant areas may be controlled temporarily with beta-rays, superficial X-rays, topical nitrogen mustard and systemic cytotoxic drugs. The end stage of the disease is a major and upsetting nursing problem,

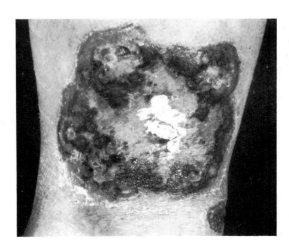

Fig. 68 Mycosis fungoides showing tumour stage and early ulceration.

just like pemphigus already described (see page 96). The use of topical potent steroids sometimes combined with phenoxyethanol 2% or econazole 0.25% and applied on spreads gives temporary ease.

The leukaemias

The leukaemias are also reticuloses which can involve the skin in the terminal stages, especially when of the lymphatic variety. Reduced immunity can result in skin infections including herpes zoster, and bruising and purpura follow platelet abnormality. The rare toxic reaction to the condition can be pruritic, bullous, exfoliative or similar to erythema multiforme.

Hodgkin's disease

Hodgkin's disease is also a reticulosis and can cause similar changes. Treatment of the leukaemias is by various combinations of cytotoxic drugs. Hodgkin's disease can be additionally treated by X-ray therapy.

Secondary malignant tumours

Secondary malignant tumours of the skin are very rare, but during the terminal stages of the illness do occur as widespread nodules, arising from primaries in the breast, uterus, stomach, kidneys or lung. Diagnosis by biopsy is very easy and should be undertaken when unusual nodules appear in patients of over 50 years of age.

Terminal care

The last few chapters have given descriptions of physical conditions that not only can be severely disabling but may also have fatal outcomes. The presence of a major illness can be very demoralising. Patients and relatives should be helped to adapt to the limitations imposed by the sickness. The social and medical aspects need sympathetic and compassionate management; the team's aim is to improve the quality of life for someone who has a skin disease that is intractable.

Terminal care can be especially distressing. Patients and relatives need the nursing and medical support and back-up mentioned towards the end of Chapter 15. The nurse must keep cheerful and ensure that the patient is clean, dry and comfortable. Even the provision of a wig is important for maintaining self-esteem and peace of mind in a patient who has lost his hair due to cytoxic drug therapy. The presence of the patient's chaplain may also help. Pain must always be relieved. As drug addiction is not a problem in a terminal illness, analgesics should be given in really adequate doses as tolerance develops. Opiates not only are excellent analgesics but help the patients become more tranquil. The patient must never feel alone. In hospital the nurse should spend as much time with him as possible; at home the relatives must do the same. In either setting the patient should be allowed peace and dignity to the end.

Chapter 17. Procedures—biopsy, therapeutic and cosmetic

Biopsy

The importance of making an accurate diagnosis from the history and characteristics of the rash has already been stressed. Sometimes the evidence is conflicting and it is necessary to take a biopsy of the skin for histological examination:

> The rash was patchy and mainly affected the trunk. Although it looked like a seborrhoeic dermatitis there was no response to treatment. It had very slowly worsened over the past decade; by now the patient was 57. Biopsy was therefore taken from the thickest patch. The pathologist was given full details of the differential diagnosis which had been listed carefully in the order of probability. He appreciated all the details, having a special interest in dermatology.
> He commented that the quantity of round-cell infiltrate just below the epidermis was far too great for a straightforward dermatitis or eczema; the patient had a premycotic eruption. Repeat biopsy half a year later substantiated the diagnosis of mycosis fungoides.

Biopsy is usually a simple procedure and patients should be reassured that the operation is a very minor one. On the other hand they must rest the part afterwards and also keep it warm and dry to obtain the minimum of scarring. Biopsies from the legs may cause ulceration if these instructions are not followed and if an elastic web bandage is not worn as an additional dressing. There is less scarring from surgery if the stitches are of the correct tension and not crowded together or left in too long; too few stitches taken out too soon may result in rupture of the wound with considerable scarring. A good compromise can be achieved by removing alternate stitches on the fourth day and the remainder on the seventh. All the stitches from facial biopsies should normally be removed on the fifth day and from the limbs on the tenth. The extra support given by adhesive strip-dressings such as 'butterfly' or 'steristrip' makes it possible to remove the sutures earlier.

Punch biopsies are quicker and easier to carry out, but do not provide such a satisfactory histological specimen as there is usually distortion and no normal skin for comparison.   An elliptical surgical incision gives the best results, and the specimen should include some normal skin from the edge of the lesion as well as the dermis to show the depth of a lesion or how far a tumour is invading. A hook is preferable to forceps as it is important to avoid trauma to the cells in the specimen, especially in some tumours such as early mycosis fungoides. Once removed the specimen should be laid on its side on blotting paper to make it easier for the pathologist to orientate it correctly for processing. Once stuck to the blotting paper the specimen should immediately be placed in a fixative.

Procedure

The biopsy trolley should firstly be swabbed with an antiseptic such as chlorhexidine 0.5% in 70% isopropylalcohol and dried off with a disposable towel. When the patient is prepared and the doctor ready to start, the sterile biopsy pack is opened by the nurse and set out on the top of the trolley. The pack may be made up as shown on page 187. The lower shelf of the trolley should contain two 2 ml disposable syringes and 25 mm/5/10 needles, an antiseptic lotion such as the chlorhexidine 0.5% in 70% isopropylalcohol or 'Mediswabs', surgical blades including the equivalent of Bard Parker size 15, Ethicon or Abrasilk with needle size 03, surgical gloves, small pieces of blotting paper about 1.5 cm by 1.5 cm, tissue fixative bottles containing 10% neutral formol saline, dry dressings, acrylic resin spray and microporous as well as extensible adhesive plaster.

Lignocaine 1% plain is probably the best local anaesthetic for histological specimens, though 2% may be needed for nerve blocks and small facial biopsies. Adrenaline when sterilised becomes acidic and this may cause swelling of the dermal collagen fibres when viewed through the microscope.

It is convenient to keep the electric cautery within easy reach, together with the various burners, as described later (page 180). This is because good cosmetic results follow excision of part of a lesion for histology, with cautery to what remains. A completed biopsy form would also be needed providing full clinical details for sending to the pathologist, including a note as to the area from where the specimen was taken. The nurse and doctor should of course have checked the patient's notes to make sure that they were operating on the right area —and person! A consent form should have already been completed.

Therapeutic and cosmetic procedures

Curettage

Curettage can be used to remove a lesion instead of excising it. This is done by a scraping action with an instrument shaped like a sharp spoon, and called a curette. The cosmetic result is better than with surgery, as there is remarkably little scarring even though large areas are attacked. The specimens are not so suitable for histological examination because they are distorted, unorientated and not attached to normal skin or the normal dermis. Curettage is excellent when the diagnosis is reasonably certain such as in the treatment of a seborrhoeic keratosis. The chunks of tissue removed provide good cytological evidence of the diagnosis. Never throw a specimen away. It is sometimes impossible to be absolutely sure of the diagnosis. The pathologist can quickly show the error so that further treatment can then be carried out. A malignant melanoma may occasionally be mistaken for a pigmented seborrhoeic keratosis.

Electric cautery

An electric cautery is a platinum wire heated by electric current which

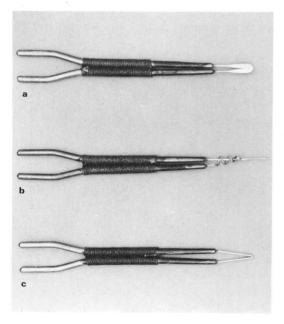

Fig. 69   Electric cautery. (a) Burner F, (b) cold-point, (c) burner S

is varied by a knob on the transformer. Several shapes are needed, as shown in Fig. 69. 65 mm is a convenient length. (Cautery burners, produced by Rimmer Brothers, London EC1R 0DD.) Cautery (burner F, Fig. 69a) is very useful to smooth down non-pigmented moles under local anaesthesia to just above the skin surface. The final contraction of the tissue then makes the area level within a few months; overtreatment produces dimples which catch the light and cause shadows, thus highlighting the defect. Any hairs coming from these non-pigmented moles must be destroyed at least 2 months before the main cauterisation is undertaken, as otherwise they may become trapped by the new epithelium and cause a foreign body reaction. The hairs can either be removed with a sharp-pointed electric cautery needle (coldpoint, Fig. 69b), or with the cosmetic diathermy needle described in the next section.

Cautery (burner S, Fig. 69c) is useful for stemming the bleeding after curettage of a pyogenic granuloma, an infectious lesion such as molluscum contagiosum, or a virus wart. All cosmetic procedures in children are much easier if they have been sedated; hydroxyzine (Atarax) given an hour beforehand has been found effective.

Diathermy

Cosmetic diathermy is best carried out with a machine primarily designed for the treatment of hirsutes by epilation. The unipolar diathermy current is transmitted to the lesion by a platinum iridium needle. On the side of the needle holder is a fine switch to control the periods of treatment without shaking the needle; the intensity of the current is altered by the dial on the machine.

Spider angiomas are easily treated with cosmetic diathermy. The needle is carefully inserted alongside the central vessel with the visual aid of a lens after firstly assessing its position by prodding with the wire of a paper clip. Electric cautery (coldpoint) pressed on the naevus and then switched on is an alternative treatment, as is the cryoprobe spray to be described later.

Cosmetic diathermy is useful for the treatment of small retention cysts on the face, known as milia. It is also the best treatment for telangiectatic areas such as the vascular lesions of adenoma sebaceum; cautery can be used to good effect on the fleshy areas, but extensive examples are best treated under general anaesthesia or by dermabrasion.

Trichloracetic acid

Trichloracetic acid, applied very accurately with a small wisp of cottonwool round the end of a wooden applicator, gives good results with · xanthomata (Fig. 70a, b) and seborrhoeic keratosis. The acid must be localised on facial lesions by putting soft paraffin round them. It produces a fine white burn while the patient experiences a stinging sensation. The white area can be controlled by further application or the use of calamine lotion to neutralise the acid. More cottonwool is needed on the applicator for the last mentioned. No local anaesthetic is needed. The acid should always be used in a saturated solution from a bottle in which there are both liquid and crystals. Keep it away from your own skin!

Phenol

Phenol is useful for cauterising the inner linings of cysts or sinuses. First, their contents are removed and then a sharpened applicator that has been soaked in the phenol is introduced, using a circular movement. There may be some initial bleeding. Pyogenic granulomas can be effectively painted with phenol and treatment continued at weekly

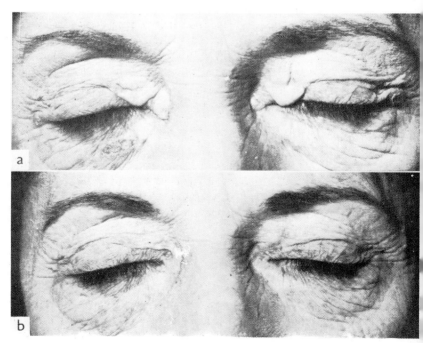

Fig. 70a & b   Xanthomata before and after treatment with trichloracetic acid.

intervals using a silver nitrate stick. Curettage and cautery gives better and quicker results; it also provides a specimen for histological confirmation of the diagnosis. This is important as a non-pigmenting malignant melanoma can occasionally look like a pyogenic granuloma.

Treatment of multiple solar keratoses

It cannot be stressed too forcefully that one must be sure of the diagnosis before attempting to destroy any lesion. The treatment of multiple solar (exposure, senile) keratoses has been revolutionised by two procedures:
1 The use of local antimitotic preparations, but a biopsy should first be carried out on any suspicious lesion.
2 Cryotherapy which has the advantage that 'frozen' specimens can be taken for histology at the same time with the aid of a curette.

1 Antimitotic creams

5-Fluorouracil 5% cream should be applied thinly and accurately twice daily to the solar keratoses. Erythema should develop after a few days followed by blistering, peeling and cracking within a fortnight. Some lesions may ulcerate and feel sore. These reactions are an index of the effectiveness of the treatment which usually has to be continued for 3–4 weeks. Transient erythema may occur on the adjacent normal skin. Pre-existing subclinical lesions may become apparent. Sunlight increases the intensity of the reaction, as does occlusion which is not normally recommended.

The cream should not be allowed to come into contact with any mucous membrane surfaces, particularly the eyes. The hands should be washed thoroughly after applying it. The total area of skin treated at any one time should not exceed 500 cm^2 (approximately 23×23 cm) as some of the drug is absorbed. Cosmetics should not be applied to the areas being treated. Severe reactions may be controlled with an intermediate strength corticosteroid cream. Healing is usually complete within 2 months.

2 Cryotherapy

Cryotherapy is quicker than 5-fluorouracil 5% cream but the cosmetic result is no better. It has the advantage over trichloracetic acid in that the depth of tissue destruction can be more readily controlled, and there tends to be less scarring. The modern machines (cryoprobe) are easier and quicker to use than cautery as local anaesthetics are rarely needed. Freezing causes cell death or injury and intravascular thrombosis, the effects being more severe at the centre of the frozen area. Inflammation begins to settle within 3 days but blistering or necrosis takes longer. Repeat freeze/thaw cycles give better results. Underlying vital vessels, nerves and tear ducts must of course be avoided!

The freezing can be produced by letting nitrous oxide expand and transferring the coldness indirectly by metal applicators of differing shapes. Liquid nitrogen is much colder and is usually available in an industrial area. The depth of freezing is difficult to control when it is applied on swabs. It is more flexible when used in a cryoprobe with the same type of metal applicators as with nitrous oxide. More convenient still is the cryoprobe jet where the liquid nitrogen can be accurately sprayed on the area to be treated.

The treatment may cause some pain but the freezing has its own anaesthetic effect. As with all minor cosmetic procedures, sedatives and analgesics help the patient tolerate the treatment more readily. The following list contains diagnoses where cryotherapy is considered the treatment of choice:

> Epidermal naevi, particularly the linear ones, pyogenic granuloma, acquired haemangioma, lentigo, malignant lentigo (intra-epidermal malignant melanoma), solar keratosis, kerato-acanthoma in the aged, intra-epidermal carcinoma (Bowen's disease), leukoplakia, mucous cysts and vascular lesions of the mouth, some basal-celled carcinomas, keloids.

CO_2 snow

Carbon dioxide (CO_2) snow is made by letting the gas under pressure expand into a collecting bag or sparklet chamber. It is not as cold as liquid nitrogen. It is applied in a stick, or as a slush, made up with a few drops of acetone. A plastic container should be used to make the last mentioned, not a metal galley pot that will remove all the cold from the slush. Nodular and pustular acne lesions do well with the slush applied on a swab to whiten the skin for up to 5 seconds each fortnight. Thicker areas should be treated with the stick for up to 10 seconds. Similar effects can be obtained by fluoromethane (Freon) local anaesthetic spray, but the patient's eyes must be protected from its accidental misdirection.

Leukoplakia, solar keratoses, non-pigmented moles, seborrhoeic keratoses or the pulsating angiomas of liver failure can usually be treated with either the carbon dioxide stick or the cryoprobe.

There is a natural overlap between surgery and dermatology in the treatment of non-malignant skin excrescences. The surgeon will probably excise a seborrhoeic keratosis while the dermatologist will curette it; multiple skin tags might be treated by the surgeon with diathermy or the dermatologist by cryoprobe. It would be equally effective if the family doctor snipped off the lesions with sharp scissors, or the nurse painted them accurately with trichloracetic acid!

Tattoos

Tattoos are due to various pigments introduced into the skin. Alcohol by mouth is the usual analgesic! Patients should be told that plastic surgery is the only way of removing them with minimal scarring. When scarring is not a problem, as in a male who wants the name of a previous girlfriend obliterated, treatment with cautery, salabrasion or even dermabrasion can be undertaken.

Salabrasion has been known since the first century AD, but there has recently been renewed interest in it for the removal of tattoos. The areas are shaved and cleaned and a local anaesthetic is given. Salabrasion is then carried out by rubbing the tattooed skin with moist sterile gauze dipped in table salt until the epidermis has gone and a uniform glistening surface is revealed. The salt is then usually rinsed off and infection minimised by applying an antiseptic cream.

Dermabrasion is now used less frequently than in previous years as some of the results were disappointing due to the scarring produced. Rhinophyma due to rosacea, port wine marks, or the pitted scarring from acne were the main conditions treated. Dermabrasion can also be used to scar over tattoos, as has been mentioned.

Hair transplantation

Hair transplantation is an expensive procedure and requires great expertise and patience, but can be of cosmetic value. It involves taking multiple punch biopsies from the posterior areas of scalp which are not expected to become bald. These hairs retain their tendency not to age. Less time-consuming is the use of punch biopsies to form a perimeter of hair, most useful to mask the gap that would otherwise be obvious between the scalp and wig.

Pinch grafting

Pinch grafting can be carried out in a clean room specifically designated for biopsies, or in a surgical theatre. It is helpful for the treatment of leg ulcers when a perfect cosmetic result is not needed (Fig. 71). The following notes are appended for general guidance. Secondary infection should first be controlled by suitable antiseptic lotions or creams such as silver nitrate 0.5% with chlorhexidine 0.2%.

Suggested pinch grafting procedure

1   Patient to be kept in bed for the 7 days prior to the operation but allowed up for toilet and washing. Physiotherapy and exercises in bed to be continued until the day before grafting. The foot of bed to be elevated to about 20°. Oxytetracycline 250 mg to be taken 4 times daily for 5 days commencing on first day.

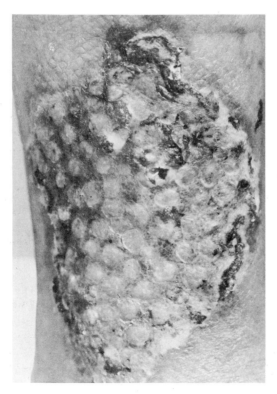

Fig. 71 Successful healing pinch graft of a gravitational ulcer 2 weeks after operation.

Checklist
Biopsy pack (see right)
Large scalpel blade
Ampoules sterile water
Hyalase ampoules
Lignocaine 1% local
25 mm cutting needles ½ circle × 4
Chlorhexidine tulle
Non-adherent dressings, large
Crêpe bandages
Zinc paste with icthammol bandages
Plaster shears (to remove icthammol)
Large paper disposal bags
Crystal violet 0.5% in water, orange
  sticks and gallipot to mark
  donor grafts
Normal saline sachets for the gallipot
A sterile bowl to contain water at
  body temperature on which floats
  a gallipot for the graft
Clinical notes
Operation consent form signed
  (doctor to explain to patient)

Biopsy pack
2 Gillies hooks (3043, 3044, 185 mm)
Pointed scissors (115 mm, 140 mm)
Kilner's needle holder (135 mm)
Scalpel holder and small blade
2 pairs mosquito forceps (130 mm)
*1 pair dissecting forceps (155 mm)
*1 curette, Lang's scoup (135 mm)

*not to be used for histology

2a When the infection is predominantly with Gram-positive organisms such as staphylococci, the ulcer to be dressed from the first day with half-strength Milton solution and liquid paraffin mixed in equal parts, applied on absorbent gauze 3 times a day for 5 days, the dressings being remoistened twice during each night.

2b For Gram-negative infections such as *Pseudomonas*, use 3-hourly soaks with gauze soaked in silver nitrate 0.5% and chlorhexidine 0.2% in water, and moistened twice at night.

3 Following this for 2 days, the ulcer to be dressed 3 times a day with gauze soaked in normal saline solution, dressings being kept continually moistened in between times as required.

4 After the operation donor sites to be dressed with several layers of chlorhexidine acetate 0.5% tulle (Bactigras) and covered with two layers of gauze.

5 The grafted area to be treated as **4**, but a zinc paste with icthammol bandage followed by a crêpe bandage is then applied. (Plaster of Paris to be used whenever patients are known to interfere with their dressings.)

6 For the first week after the operation the patient to be allowed out of bed only for toilet, and when doing so must walk keeping the ankle stiff.

7 Bed rest elevation to be continued. Bandages to be removed on seventh day by the doctor, and daily dressings carried out with the chlorhexidine tulle by nursing staff.

8 Physiotherapy to be recommenced and exercises gradually reintroduced from the seventh day after the operation.

9 If secondary infection develops, swab to be taken for culture and local treatment changed to silver nitrate 0.5% with chlorhexidine 0.2% in cetamacragol A cream as required.

Insight

In any cosmetic procedure it is important that the patient's reasons for seeking treatment are carefully assessed. In some instances the disfigurement is obvious. In others the defect may be slight, but the patient blames it for feelings of inferiority or failure; in other words, anxiety from quite a different source is projected on to the minor blemish. No cosmetic procedures, however perfect, will ever satisfy these patients who are often the bane of the plastic surgeon's life. One should treat the symptoms first and only afterwards attend to the cosmetic defect.

Chapter 18. Investigations— histological, mycological and bacteriological

Histology

The careful taking of a specimen of tissue for histological examination has been mentioned in Chapter 17. The lesion selected should be an early one and typical of the rash. Blisters should be removed intact and must not be more than 24 hours old. After orientation the specimen is placed in fixative to prevent degenerative changes taking place. A 10% solution of neutral formalin in saline may be used, but glutaraldehyde is more popular for electron microscopy. Once processed and embedded in wax the tissue is sliced very thinly by a microtome. One of the slices is then placed on a microscope slide and stained so that the cells, nuclei, and different fibres can be seen by the different colours they take up. Fat dissolves out in the processing, so when fat stains are needed the pathology form should be boldly marked to prevent the specimen being put through the routine processing as soon as it is received at the laboratory. Communication between all members of the team here extends to the pathologist and his technicians. This is by means of the pathology forms which must be correctly filled in. An even better method is to staple to the form a copy of the clinical letter that has been sent to the family doctor. This letter usually gives the reasons for the investigation in much greater detail than is possible on a form, and taking an extra carbon copy takes no time at all.

Tissue for direct immunofluorescence should be frozen in carbon dioxide snow, and sent to laboratories specialising in this investigation. Serum for indirect immunofluorescence should not be frozen.

Mycology

Mycology is needed to prove the diagnoses of the various fungus infections. Fungicidal preparations should not have been used for a week before the specimens are taken. Pieces of affected nails can easily be obtained with sharp scissors or clippers. Epilation forceps should be used to remove infected hairs. Specimens are taken from the skin by scraping with a blunt scalpel. The active edge of a lesion but particularly the roof of a blister gives the greatest number of positive results. One part is placed in warmed potassium hydroxide 10% on a microscope slide and examined for fungal filaments. These usually branch at right angles with the exception of pityriasis versicolor where the branches are Y shaped. Candida can be recognised when budding and the corynebacteria of erythrasma can be seen with the oil immersion lens. The other part of the specimen is placed on special culture media, and incubated for at least 3 weeks. Certain laboratories specialise in these examinations, and specimens can be sent to them by post if they are wrapped in black paper to make them easy to see. Reports of the microscopy are available within a few days but culture may take up to a month. Make sure the patient does not make an unnecessary journey to the doctor, only to find that the report is not yet available.

Bacteriology

Bacteriology is necessary to identify the causative organism of a pyogenic infection. It is also important in the treatment of severe infections where the organism must be sensitive to antibiotics that are being given systemically:

> He was a severe diabetic who had attended the clinic for many years. He was now 53. A carbuncle had developed on the back of his neck and had spread to measure 6 cm in diameter. It throbbed and was tender. It hadn't localised like an ordinary boil, the surrounding skin being inflamed and swollen. Swabs were taken from its edge as well as the pus, and an antibiotic given that was usually effective against the staphylococcus commonly encountered in the hospital at that time. The patient was then admitted and treated locally with crystal violet 0.5% in water twice daily. The bacteriology report showed that the staphylococcus was sensitive to the antibiotic given but resistant to penicillin. Healing was slow but uneventful. Control of the diabetes was most troublesome particularly at the height of the infection.

Routine bacteriology is useful in the management of leg ulcers to check on the quantity of organisms present and to see if one is predominant, so that suitable antiseptic creams can be given. Bacteriology is also needed before pinch grafting. The antibiotic sensitivity pattern should only be asked for when there is a clinical need; laboratory resources are not unlimited, particularly with regard to the technician's time.

Swabs dry out during the delay between being taken and being plated on the culture media in the laboratory. This may kill off some organisms, especially *Pseudomonas*. The use of liquid transport media such as Stuart's may therefore be necessary. The swab should be moistened with the liquid if the lesion is dry, rubbed on to it, and then broken off into the media bottle. If the cap is screwed on firmly to keep out air (and other contaminants) then anaerobic culture can also be undertaken.

Nasal and perineal swabs should be taken when the infection is predominantly around these areas and when carriage of *Staphylococcus pyogenes* is suspected. Recurrent or chronic infection may be due to carriage of organisms by another member of the family who will also need investigating.

Virology

Virology may be necessary in systemic illness, for example in widespread infection with herpes simplex (cold sores); encephalitis due to this virus is rare but does occur and can be fatal.

One method of virus identification is from monitoring any changes in specific antibody titres in the serum. Blood specimens are taken as soon as possible, at 2 weeks, and sometimes at 6 weeks. Increases in the titres are diagnostic for the specific virus in question.

Isolation or indirect identification of the virus is possible from skin lesions. This can be carried out by growing them in a culture of living cells and by electron microscopy. Scrapings or swabs can be transported between slides and vesicle fluid in a capillary tube sealed at both ends with plasticine. Some viruses are killed by drying, so swabs should also be sent in 'virus transport medium'. Unlike Stuart's, this medium needs to be kept frozen until it is required for use.

Chapter 19. PUVA, X- and Grenz-ray therapy, physiotherapy, chiropody, dietetics

A variety of therapeutic methods in dermatology utilise some form of radiation. In the electromagnetic spectrum the type of radiation depends on the wavelength. An indication is given below of the various radiations and their relative wavelengths.

Radio waves	Microwaves radar	Infra- red	Visible light	Ultraviolet A.B.C.	Grenz rays	X-rays	Gamma rays

Longer ◄─────────────── Wavelength ───────────────► Shorter

Ultraviolet radiation

The conventional mercury vapour lamp produces a lot of radiation in the mid UV range known as UVB. These rays are the cause of sunburn. In dermatology they are utilised in the treatment of acne as well as to encourage growth in indolent bed sores or leg ulcers. The amount of light falling on the skin decreases with the square of the distance from the lamp; the amount is also proportional to the exposure time. Patients must wear UV-absorbing goggles and the operators dark glasses. Physiotherapists usually give the treatment.

A new kind of treatment is now available for psoriasis called PUVA. This stands for Psoralen plus UVA (ultraviolet light A, also known as black light). Banks of fluorescent tubes either surround a cabinet in which the patient stands, or are in a canopy that comes over them on a couch. The fluorescent tubes are coated on the inside to produce the chosen wavelength. Provision should be made for the patient to be able to switch off the treatment if he gets too hot or feels faint. The amount of light given is carefully regulated, the machine switching itself off at the end of the exposure. A fair-skinned individual will not tolerate as much light as a dark one, and the dose is adjusted accordingly. Someone giving a history of always burning and never tanning in the sun would only tolerate less than a third of the initial dose of someone who never burns and always tans. Alternatively the patient's sensitivity can be determined by photo-patch testing after oral psoralen. The UVA dose is usually increased by about 25% each week, provided only mild erythema develops; this is at its maximum 3–5 days after exposure. Greater increases can be made as tolerance develops. This is due to the ensuing pigmentation which protects the skin but delays improvement. The existing pigment in the darker races is the reason why they do not do as well with PUVA treatment.

8-Methoxypsoralen causes less pigmentation than most other psoralens and is the one that is usually used. They are extracted from a weed in the *Umbilliferae* family that grows in the Nile delta. Members of this family have already been described on page 81 as being capable of causing photosensitivity dermatitis. Combining the drug with UVA is known as photochemotherapy. With energy from UVA the psoralen is bound by a photochemical reaction to DNA, the basic component of chromosomes. This inhibits epidermal synthesis of DNA and therefore epidermal turnover. In psoriasis the turnover is increased tenfold; reducing this effects clearance. Dithranol works similarly except that the energy from the UVA is not needed. PUVA is also effective in the treatment of *Mycosis fungoides* where the increased cellular turnover is due to low-grade malignancy.

The methoxypsoralen can either be given systemically, as is mainly undertaken in the USA and UK, or applied locally as advocated in Germany.

Local treatment has the advantage of only affecting the area where it is applied. Complications from the treatment, to be discussed later, would thereby be reduced. Local treatment on the other hand is more time-consuming and more difficult to control. The pigmentation is greater where the psoralen is applied and therefore may be patchy and unsightly. For maximum effect the psoralen should be applied at least an hour before the UVA is given. With oral treatment the gap should be between 2 and 3 hours, the dosage depending on the weight of the patient.

Since it takes up to a day for the drug to be excreted, patients have to avoid sunlight, including that through glass, for at least this period as it is not yet known how long the drug remains in the lens. The eyes need protection with polarised sunglasses with side pieces and UV-absorbing grey or green plastic lenses to prevent the development of conjunctivitis, cataracts or retinitis. Operators should also wear these glasses. Patients must wear UV-absorbing goggles for the actual exposure, and try to keep the lids closed. The eyes should be examined before PUVA is given, and those with lens damage not treated systemically. Immediate complications from the treatment include nausea or gastric discomfort; these can be reduced by insisting that milk and a biscuit is taken with the tablet, or the dose is split and half taken half an hour beforehand. Erythema, pruritus and a feeling of the skin being tight are signs of overtreatment. Blistering rarely occurs, though it is an occasional problem with local treatment. Pruritus is more common, and can be relieved by bland emollients and antihistamines by mouth such as chlorpheniramine.

Some long-term side-effects are expected so the treatment should not be used indiscriminately. It is known that soldiers who sunbathed for long periods during the North African campaign had an increased incidence of squamous-cell carcinoma 10–20 years later. Basal-cell carcinomas are more common on exposed sites such as the face. The incidence of malignant melanoma is also increased by sun exposure. The UVA plus psoralens may have similar effects. They are expected to age the skin prematurely.

It is not yet known if the psoralens themselves can cause mutations and lead to an increased incidence of internal malignancy. Teratogenicity is a theoretical possibility, so PUVA should not be given to pregnant women.

In conclusion, the treatment can be considered clean and effective but has the disadvantage that patients have to attend special centres, and long-term side-effects are possible. It should ideally be used for older patients with severe, disabling psoriasis. The amount of treatment can be considerably reduced if PUVA is used as an addition to the dithranol regime.

The treatments described in this chapter are often adjuncts to other dermatological therapies and are given by ancillary members of the team. How can they check that the patient is carrying out the rest of the treatment unless they know what should be happening? A convenient way of doing this is for their instructions to be written up on the copy of the report that is sent to the family doctor.

X-rays

X-rays (and to a lesser extent Grenz rays) penetrate more deeply than ultraviolet light. They have a less subtle effect, usually causing cellular death. Nerves and local lymphocytes are sensitive to the rays which cause a temporary reduction of skin irritation and immunological reaction. Because of long-term complications, such as carcinogenesis, internally and externally, and damage from faulty techniques, the treatment has largely been superseded by Grenz rays. It is still used in conjunction with other therapies for chronic paronychia, certain keloids, and eczema of the hands and feet in older persons.

Grenz rays

Grenz rays only penetrate the epidermis and are therefore safer than X-rays. Even so, it is still wise to reserve the treatment for older persons. Their effect is temporary, so they must only be used as an adjunct to full dermatological therapy. They are useful to reduce the sensitivity of the skin while stronger local treatments, such as dithranol, are being introduced. Large areas can be treated using the technique of multiple 'open fields' (Figs. 72 and 73). Grenz rays have a similar effect on psoralens to that of UVA. They have a future therefore when given with psoralens for the treatment of areas such as flexures and feet that are not reached by UVA lamps. They penetrate more than UVA and

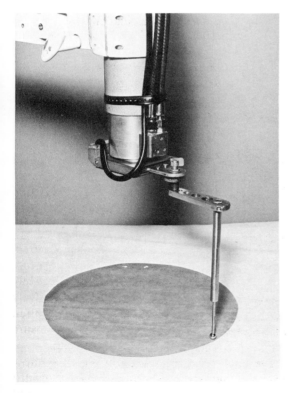

Fig. 72 End of Grenz-ray tube, showing distance piece and celluloid marker covering the areas which would be affected by the rays using the 'open field' technique.

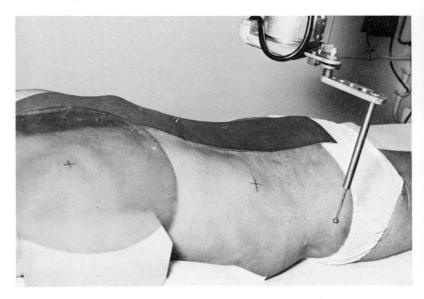

Fig. 73   Grenz ray 'open field' technique being used on a patient whose exfoliative psoriasis is clearing; the centre of each field is marked by a cross, and with calculated overlapping, widespread areas can be treated.

are useful for *Mycosis fungoides*. Grenz rays are usually effective in reducing the frequency of recurrent attacks of herpes simplex.

Physiotherapy

Physiotherapy is particularly important in dermatology in the treatment of leg ulcers, as has been mentioned on page 148. Movement must be encouraged. This entails teaching a spectrum of exercises ranging from those to undertake in bed, how to keep the feet and legs constantly moving when inadvertently having to stand, to the correction of bad walking habits. Ulcers can be painful, so activity is reduced, particularly at the ankle; the muscle pump then works less effectively and the ulcer worsens. The exercises should therefore be progressively introduced until walking is perfect. Much encouragement is often needed and the role of the nurse here is very important indeed to ensure that the exercises are being correctly carried out.

Bisgaard's massage can also be given in addition to physiotherapy. It aims to disperse oedema via the lymphatics and veins, by upward movements, particularly around the ankles. Eczematous areas should not be massaged. High elevation of the limbs for half an hour can also be carried out to reduce oedema.

Chiropody

Chiropody is needed to pare down painful callouses that interfere with walking and therefore the muscle pump. Thickened nails (onychogryphosis) can be ground down remarkably effectively by a chiropody drill. The hyperkeratotic nails in psoriasis can be treated in this way. The obese and aged may not be able to cut their toenails so regular attention may be needed.

Diabetics have to be particularly careful with their feet as sepsis may be followed by gangrene. This is because of deficient nerve and arterial supply and the well-known tendency to sepsis; all these factors delay healing. Thickened nails and callouses must therefore be treated in the early stages and an antiseptic cream such as dibromopropamidine applied for a while afterwards. Chiropody should be undertaken much more cautiously in diabetics, as has been mentioned. This also applies to arteriosclerotic limbs, or when there is nerve disease such as peripheral neuritis or paraplegia. Self-medication with salicylic acid plasters should be avoided in all these conditions; the nerve disease may make it impossible for the patient to feel that anything is wrong until it is too late.

Dietetics

Dietetics have their greatest importance in dermatology in the management of gravitational ulcers. This is because obesity is associated with immobility and poor venous return. Obese patients tend to neglect their treatment. But they don't neglect to eat, and they usually go for the wrong sorts of food too! Next time you are in a café watch what people choose and the amount consumed. Those taking salads, vegetables and proteins are usually healthy. Those taking carbohydrates are obese and pear-shaped; they follow the doggerel:

Food glorious food; whether it's boiled or stewed;
As long as it can be chewed; food glorious food.

By all means tell obese patients that there is nothing so fattening as food, but do not deride them. First find out why they are fat, tell them they will not get better until they lose weight, then explain how they should recover their health. Dieting then is just symptomatic treatment; finding the cause is more fundamental.

Most obesity is due to eating more food that the body requires. The excess is deposited as fat. The first essential is to help the patient understand why he is obese. It may become obvious that the overeating has been a straightforward habit, often since childhood or following a change of active to sedentary work. It may also reveal that his hunger is due to a psychological nervous state, which makes him yearn for the satisfying sensation of eating tasty foods.

Habits and prejudices are not easy to change. Some patients prefer to lose weight by simply reducing the amount they eat. Most, however, feel hungry with this method. Satisfying that empty feeling depends much more on the bulk of the food than its calorific value. Patients should therefore be allowed as much of the high-fibre foods as they want since they contain few calories relative to their bulk. Raw or undercooked vegetables as well as salads are therefore recommended. They can be made quite palatable if suitably flavoured with garlic, peppers and other herbs. Wine or cider vinegar freshly mixed with equal quantities of corn or soya oil makes an excellent vinaigrette. Equal quantities only should be allowed as the oil contains many calories. Do not let your patients cheat and take bread or other carbohydrates at the same time.

It is not often realised that leafy vegetables contain up to 30% protein if water is excluded from the calculation. They also contain the essential fatty acids needed for nutrition. Paperback cookery books on the preparation of salads and vegetables are easily obtainable. Some study of the French or Chinese methods of cooking vegetables would be very rewarding, but the amount of cooking oil should be kept to a minimum. Do not forget that tasting while cooking and nibbling between meals can lead to the consumption of a considerable number of calories!

Bread, bread substitutes, buns, biscuits, pastries and alcohol are high-energy foods which should be stopped or drastically reduced. Avoiding foods made with flour is a neat way of putting it! The sugars, dairy and animal fats which give most of the tempting cooking flavours should also be reduced. These may play a part in causing coronary thrombosis. The better quality soft margarines can be substituted for butter and lard, and vegetable oil used for frying. Artificial sweeteners can be taken when a sweet taste is still desired. Treatment for obesity with tablets to reduce appetite has no lasting benefit, and can produce unfortunate side-effects.

Regular exercise is an excellent way to keep healthy and also uses up some excess food; care is needed not to eat more afterwards as no weight will then be lost. It is better to eat much smaller meals, even if they are taken slightly more frequently.

Sufferers from acne and also rosacea should reduce the amount of animal and dairy fats they take. This is because these solid fats probably affect the composition of the sebum on the skin. They can use the softer margarines or the polyunsaturated oils such as corn, soya or sunflower. Acne patients should stop eating chocolate until the condition has greatly improved. Rosacea sufferers should avoid stimulants such as tea, coffee and alcohol as these dilate the facial vessels.

Alcohol consumption should be drastically reduced in patients suffering from eczema and psoriasis, as the vasodilation increases irritation and therefore encourages scratching. Weaker drinks can be allowed with food when reduction is difficult. Sudden cessation of heavy drinking is followed by irritability, sleeplessness, and sometimes hallucinations, delusions or delirium. Ward staff should remember this possibility whenever there is a change of character in a patient, particularly during the first week of admission.

Cholesterol deposits (xanthomata) in the skin can be caused by excessive consumption of dairy and animal fats and occasionally sugars. The deposits are important markers of internal disease as they also occur in vital vessels of the heart and brain. There are many other causes of these diseases which must be fully investigated and treated. Diabetes and familial hypercholesterosis are just two examples.

Allergy to gluten in wheat flour is a cause of gluten enteropathy. This is a condition associated with dermatitis herpetiformis, as mentioned on page 94. Urticaria can be due to allergy to certain foods, as mentioned on page 70. Food preservatives, dyes, and even the colour of medicinal tablets can cause problems. Elimination diets are sometimes helpful in proving the diagnosis. The patient is given glucose and water until the rash settles. Different preparations are then added separately at 2-day intervals until the offending antigen is found. With cooperative patients the dietician may be able to do this at out-patient clinics.

The patient's motivation is all-important; dieting is no exception:

'I never eat anything doctor, just the occasional cup of tea.' Being accustomed to patients expecting you to believe the impossible, or more correctly what they do not want to face up to, is part of medicine. A list was prepared of this patient's typical day's eating and drinking. Most of the calories came from approximately a loaf of bread a day! Admission to hospital with dieting was suggested to heal her chronic leg ulcer. She looked horrified but later consented. The dietician arranged a reducing diet. There was a slight gain in weight. The diet was halved, and the nurses tested the urine to exclude ketosis. Still there was no change. The charge nurse arranged photography of the ulcer in another part of the hospital group. When the ward lockers were spring-cleaned, the door was opened and several items fell to the floor—all ham sandwiches!

Chapter 20. The dermatology team

Specialisation in medicine has had to develop, as it is impossible for one single discipline to encompass all the known advances. Dermatology is a fascinating subject as there is an interesting overlap with all other specialities:

> She was an American visiting George Washington's ancestral home in Lancashire, and went to the local family doctor for her repeat depot steroid injection. He happened to be a member of the dermatology team at the local hospital, and was interested in the number of experts she had already seen. The oral surgeon and the hair specialist had prescribed local steroids and referred her to a gynaecologist, who recommended addition of the depot injections. The lesions in the mouth, scalp and vulva were all due to the one condition—lichen planus.

It does not matter which specialist is responsible for a patient's cure. What is invaluable is that they all work together and do not lose the patient's trust by giving differing opinions.

Medical and nursing etiquette developed at a time when opium and laxatives were virtually the only specific treatments. The physician's effectiveness then was mainly due to placebo response, faith and suggestion. Placebos are biologically inert substances, but during their use the patient believes that he is receiving some special treatment. It is equally important that the doctor and nurse communicate faith and enthusiasm to the patient. It is here that their personalities have the greatest impact.

The ward sister's faith in a particular tranquilliser is as important for the smooth running of her psychiatric ward as the specific effectiveness of the drug; introducing a placebo without her knowledge results in little initial change in the patient's condition. This is quite salutary, and makes one wonder how much of what we believe today to be specific treatment will be shown in later years just to have been placebo response.

The effectiveness of any treatment that depends upon faith and suggestion can very easily be destroyed by a snide comment. The need for unanimity amongst the team is now even more important with the greater number of staff involved. All members should communicate freely with each other but within the team and following the guidelines of the International Code of nursing ethics. The need for this communication is well illustrated by the duties, to be described, of the medical social workers and occupational health and community nurses.

Medical social workers

Medical social workers are not just responsible for arranging convalescence or long-stay accommodation! They should be an integral part of the team's therapeutic effectiveness. This involves helping to assess the background problems and then giving temporary support while the patient can readjust to his environment. They can visit soon after breakfast and see the state of the home, the chaos of wet nappies all over the place, or the tidiness and cleanliness even when there is poverty. Confidences should only be written down with the patient's permission, and these records kept separate in locked files. It is always useful to have some reference to the existence of this confidential information in the general notes, so that the subject can be gently reintroduced if the rash does not clear up satisfactorily.

Occupational health nurse

The occupational health nurse does not merely give out aspirins! Many workers come to her just for advice and much sickness can then be averted. Sometimes she refers a patient to the family doctor or, if the problem is occupational, to the medical officer. Patients tend to talk about their jobs and the dangers involved while a cut is being dressed or a bandage applied. The nurse then is the 'eyes and ears' of the medical officer who can arrange for any risks or difficulties to be eliminated. This should include checking for safety or for the avoidance of contact with potential sensitisers, whether by the use of extractor fans, splash guards, gloves or protective clothing. It would also include transferring someone already sensitised to a different part of the factory so that contact could be avoided. Enabling a patient to continue at work is one of the best contributions the nurse can make. She will do the dressings before the employee starts work, repeating them as necessary; she will also check that he avoids other irritants until after the skin is entirely clear and, above all, warn him that his skin will not recover its general resilience for at least half a year after the rash has gone.

The word 'dermatitis' is greatly feared and it is important that the team convince the patient that the rash can be cleared. Confidence based on a full knowledge of the occupational and therapeutic situation is needed. The nurse or the social worker should be prepared to telephone the personnel manager to make sure that a man's job is not at stake if he remains away from work until the rash is totally clear. This is very important. It is well known that the prognosis in dermatitis is worse if the rash is longstanding. What is not generally realised is that all the skin must return to normal, including any dry, cracked bits between the fingers, before chronicity can be prevented.

Community nurses

Community nurses are even more in touch with patients in their homes than the doctors with whom they are working. The daily dressing of a leg ulcer will give her an opportunity for regular personal discussion with the patient to relieve his anxiety. She can also see the home surroundings and how the patient either copes or reacts to them. Some eczematous eruptions can be rapidly brought under control with daily dressings in the home environment. Once the patient has learned the treatment and improvement has started, he can continue to attend a surgery (office) or clinic periodically until the rash has gone.

Dermatology teams should cover both the physical and the psychological aspects of their patient's problems. Since patients are individuals with differing personalities they may talk more readily to one team member than to another, to a married person, to someone older or younger, or of their own sex. Members of the team also have different personalities and some find it easier to establish rapport than others. In any event the discussion should always be held in private and without interruption. The fact that the nurse is often privileged to know the patient's innermost thoughts, whether by confidences or by her observation, gives great responsibility. The need for professional discretion cannot be overemphasised. There must also be real caring, never criticism; hold the mirror to aid understanding, never point the finger of scorn.

Consultant psychiatrist

Help from the consultant psychiatrist may be needed if the patient is unresponsive. His ability to take histories or use hypnosis to reveal relevant stress may be of great value. Abreaction is also a useful procedure. This technique uses partial anaesthesia during which the patient is actively led and encouraged to relive the relevant traumatic incidents in his past. During these periods he actually believes the events are taking place, and much emotional energy is released. Support can then be given while he readjusts and recovers. Patients tend to be afraid of psychiatry, either because of its associations with mental disorders or the truths it might reveal. Careful preparation should therefore be given before they are referred.

Group psychotherapy

Group psychotherapy may be of benefit. Whereas the discussion is led by the consultant or social worker, it is the patients who contribute and question each other. Those with the same diagnosis are encouraged to discuss their problems, whether physical or emotional. For example, it is of practical benefit for patients suffering from psoriasis of the scalp simply to know the names of hairdressers who are willing to cut their hair. The discussion of an emotional problem may not only release stress but also restore balance and perspective.

Mention should be made of dermatological organisations, such as the Psoriasis and Eczema Associations, that provide help, guidance, and collect funds for research.

In the preceding two chapters many specialised techniques have been summarised which are part of a complete dermatology service. Mention has been made of the need for good communication and loyalty between team members. It goes without saying that it would then be difficult for one team member to be played against another, a ploy sometimes attempted by an upset patient:

The ward was effectively administered. Admissions were often arranged by telephone to give patients plenty of notice and make sure the time was convenient for them. The twice-weekly main ward rounds were in the morning, so that patients would be left untreated for the minimum period of time. All members of the team joined in the discussion afterwards and contributed to solving the problems that had been encountered.

One man's admission was necessitated by a flare-up of his eczema after he had been declared redundant at the age of 42, but he had had the rash since getting married 4 years previously. He was aggressive with the others in the ward and complained about the food, which was unusual as it was considered the best in the hospital group. The consultant commented on the burnished appearance of his rash. The retort was, 'It's due to the nurses taking off the dressings. Your treatment's no use so they are trying something else.' This was all untrue, so the social worker was asked to find out what was upsetting him. It was only after making a special visit to the home that she found the answer; the wife confided that her husband had always been impotent.

It has been shown that there must always be loyalty and good communication in a dermatology team. The enthusiasm and happiness with which members work together sets the tone of the team. At all times there must be meticulous attention to detail, whether physical or psychological, as in no other way can chronicity be prevented.

Chapter 21. Structure, function and care of the skin, nails and hair

Would you have read as far as this if this book had started with the structure of the skin? Being a subject difficult to make interesting, it has been left almost until the end. But it is as well to refresh your knowledge of this amazing organ and tell you more about its function and care.

Structure and function of skin, nails and hair

Fig. 74 shows a cross-section of normal skin. Superficially there is the horny layer which is protective and contains a basket-weave of keratin. It is formed from the prickle-celled layer which comes next, these two comprising the epidermis. Then comes the dermis containing collagen fibres, the 'leather' which gives the skin its strength. Amongst the fibres are blood vessels, cutaneous nerves, lymphatics, sweat glands (10) and hair follicles (3) with their surrounding sebaceous glands (4). The deepest layer contains the subcutaneous fat tissue, together with more collagen.

Pigment cells offer protection against ultraviolet light. They are found in the basal layer of the epidermis, and occur in the same number in the 'white' and 'dark' skinned races; it is the differing quantity of melanin pigment the cells synthesise that determines the colour. Lack of protective pigmentation is the reason for the increased incidence of malignancy in fair-skinned individuals in the tropics.

Just under the epidermis is a folded plexus of capillaries associated with the ridges on the skin called 'dermatoglyphics'; those on the hands are known as 'fingerprints'. Nerves and their endings are present in the plexus. Nerves also supply the hair follicles and the specialised touch organs known as Pacinian bodies (7).

The epidermis is formed from the outer layer of the developing embryo known as ectoderm. Nervous tissue, as has been mentioned on page 7, is derived from an infolding of this same ectoderm. Comment has already been made about the very close relationship that exists between skin and nerves. This is what one would expect as, from the

205

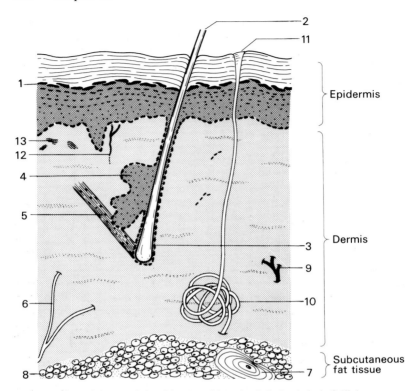

Fig. 74 Constituents of the skin. 1, epidermis; 2, hair; 3, hair follicle;
4, sebaceous gland; 5, muscle fibres of M. arrector pili; 6, blood vessel;
7, Pacinian body; 8, fat lobules; 9, cutaneous nerve; 10, sweat glands; 11, sweat
duct opening; 12, terminal nerve fibrils; 13, collagen bundles.

early stages of single-cell evolution, the skin has acted as the main
organ of touch and contact with the outer world. Later the eyes and
ears developed to give more distant contact; their outer parts are
derived from ectoderm, also by a process of infolding. Hair and nails
are evolved from the horny layer of the epidermis by a similar process.
The relationship of the hair (2) to its follicle (3) can be seen in Fig. 74.

In animals the hair and fur have protective and thermoregulatory
functions. The first mentioned is not so important now for man since
he has developed the ability to clothe himself. Heat regulation is also
controlled by nerves affecting blood flow in the great subepidermal
network of capillaries and the activity of the sweat glands.

As well as receiving stimuli, the skin and appendages are important
organs of expression. Think of the fluttered eyelid, the dilated pupil in

enjoyment, the flush of emotion, the smile of real joy! And the skin feels so much warmer during these moments. Then there are all the many ways in which the skin expresses itself in times of illness, as has been shown in this book. One not mentioned is that the hair can stand on end with fear; the actual muscles that do this are shown at (5) in Fig. 74.

Care of skin, nails and hair

Care of the nurse's skin, hair and nails is important, not only for personal reasons but also because she is the team's main ambassador. The normal skin remains greased and hydrated by sebum and the water it retains. It protects the individual from chemicals, bacterial assault, heat and cold. Frequent washing, strong detergents, spirits or antiseptics degrease the skin, rendering it vulnerable and liable to develop dermatitis, as has been stressed on page 82. Do not forget that an attack could alter your whole career and homelife, so take care. Scrubbing the skin is not good for it. After handling a dirty problem, it is best to wash the hands with a good quality toilet soap and dry them with cotton towelling. Then without fail apply an emollient cream to the skin and nails, as the degreasing mentioned earlier causes flaking or splitting nails, which is a chapping effect from dehydration.

Care of the hair and scalp go hand in hand with caring about one's personal appearance. Those with greasy scalps need to shampoo more frequently than those with dry ones. A good quality detergent shampoo is recommended. Normally this will take place once a week or fortnight. Strong brushing or scalp massage is a waste of time. Dandruff can usually be controlled by increasing the frequency of shampooing or using one that is medicated. On occasion it may be necessary to resort to the treatments for pityriasis capitis, mentioned on page 61.

There is no doubt that pityriasis and psoriasis encourage hair loss, so treatment must be thorough. On the other hand there is natural hair loss related to a replacement process. Hairs have a prolonged growth phase at a rate of a centimetre per month and lasting about 3 years. This is followed by a resting phase of roughly 3 months when the hair is shed. Hair shedding therefore is normal. Unfortunately the over-anxious or overattentive may interpret this as hair disease and need reassuring accordingly.

Nurses are sometimes asked about permanent waving of the hair. All the processes, whether the seldom-used hot method or the cold perm, are irritants to the scalp. At least a fortnight should elapse therefore after an attack of pityriasis capitis or eczema before the hair is permed. Until then curlers or rollers at night can be used so that the patient is happy and confident with her appearance. The cold perm process employs thioglycolate to soften the hair which is then wound around curlers. A neutraliser is applied about 30 minutes later and the hair will then remain curled. The thioglycolate should be kept off the forehead, neck and scalp with strips of cottonwool. It must be quickly neutralised and a shampoo used if there is a sensation of burning. Sometimes the hair may have previously been weakened by bleaching, and despite correct perming techniques the curls come off in chunks! The alopecia is not of course permanent.

Like all medical specialities, dermatology has its own descriptive terms, most of them having Latin or Greek origins. Alopecia, for instance, comes from the Greek word for 'fox mange'. A short glossary follows, listing the more important terms that will be encountered during discussion and when dipping into reference books.

Glossary

Macule. small non-elevated area of a different colour
Papule. small circumscribed solid elevation of the skin
Nodule. small circumscribed protuberance or lump
Vesicle. small localised blister in the skin
Pustule. a vesicle containing pus
Bulla. a blister roofed with all or part of the epidermis, usually over 1 cm diameter

Atrophy. wasting
Burrows. seen in scabies
Circinate. having a circular outline or ring formation
Comedone. the same as a blackhead, which is a dilated sebaceous gland and blocked hair follicle
Crusting. dried serum
Cyst. a sac
Erythema. redness
Fissure. crack
Hypertrophy. increase in thickness
Keratosis. horny thickening
Lichenification. thickening
Livedo. a bluish discolouration of the skin
Pigment. staining
Plaque. an elevated area of skin affection
Purpura. haemorrhage into the skin as petechiae or macules
Reticulate. net like
Scaling. sheets of horny cells
Telangiectasia. a network of dilated capillary blood vessels
Ulcer. a loss of epithelium
Weeping. oozing of serum
Wheal. transient swelling of the skin without scaling

Chapter 22. Principles of physical treatment and preparations to avoid

The different treatments that the consultant or family doctor prescribe can be a fascinating study. The basic medicaments are chosen for their chemical and physical activity, but the minor variations between preparations are much more subtle. Not only experience of their mode of action is important, but there must be knowledge of the conditions allowing for their maximum effect. The art of therapeutics comes mainly from experience either personal or from one's teachers, since much of dermatology is learned on the apprenticeship basis.

The importance of prescribing and carrying out treatment with confidence has already been stressed. This is impossible without full knowledge of the medicament. It is better to learn all about a few preparations than a little about many. Ingram taught *'Be master of your own method'*. Regimes should be simple; General Eisenhower is reported to have said that if a battle plan would not go on a postcard the battle would be lost!

Formularies are rationalised lists of treatment. Rationalisation encourages simplicity and therefore safety; it is also convenient for dispensing and application. The formulary given in the Appendix is one of personal choice, but is also based on clinical evaluation. It lists a few basic necessities for a dermatology service. These have been taken from various official formularies, so that the preparations would be standardised and readily available in the scattered part of the Lake District that the unit covers. The dithranol (anthralin) ointment prescriptions were developed locally. Most details of worldwide prescriptions can be obtained from Martindale's *Extra Pharmacopoeia*, as well as full notes of their advantages and possible side-effects.

The choice of a medicament depends of course on its physical action. The strength used is sometimes critical. For example, silver nitrate is a good antiseptic for Gram-negative organisms at about 0.5% strength, but above 1% it acts as an astringent or caustic and coagulates proteins.

The base in which a medicament is applied is equally important. Pastes consist of powders, usually mixed in soft paraffin; ointments are greasier as they contain less powder. Pastes, being stiffer, are more protective and better for the treatment of dry and thicker eruptions. They allow natural healing to take place underneath them. Lotions are fluid preparations; they have a cooling effect due to evaporation and are suitable for the treatment of wet rashes. Creams contain oils and water together with an emulsifier and can be applied to either moist or dry rashes. They are popular with patients as they are pleasant to use. The acceptability of a preparation is all important. For example, ointments are more effective than creams mainly because of their greater depot effect; but because they are greasier there is less chance of the patient carrying out the treatment satisfactorily, unless the therapeutic advantage is carefully explained.

The degree of activity of an eruption determines the choice of medicament, its strength and the base or vehicle that would be most suitable for the particular occasion. An acute exudative rash would only tolerate a bland and soothing lotion or cream, whereas one which is chronic or indolent would respond best to strong ointments or pastes. Figure 75 shows the relationship between the pathological phase of activity of the rash and the base and strength of the medicament best suited for its treatment.

It is wiser to err on the side of simplicity and use bland preparations rather than complicated or strong ones. In many instances the skin only needs protection while natural healing takes place. Frequent changes in the choice of medicament only complicate management. It takes a few days for most preparations to show that they are working. If a change is made too soon it is then not possible to know which medicament is responsible for either a response or a treatment reaction.

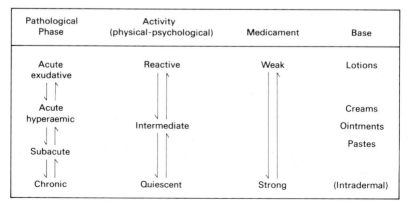

Pathological Phase	Activity (physical-psychological)	Medicament	Base
Acute exudative	Reactive	Weak	Lotions
Acute hyperaemic	Intermediate		Creams
			Ointments
			Pastes
Subacute			
Chronic	Quiescent	Strong	(Intradermal)

Fig. 75   How treatment is chosen to suit the state of the skin condition.

Lotions, creams or eyedrops contain water and are readily contaminated by organisms such as *Pseudomonas aeruginosa*. This may occur during manufacture but is more common during use. Patients should therefore be provided with their own pack of a medicament, creams being tubed when possible. Ointments and pastes contain no water and rarely cause cross infection. Even so, nurses using them from stock containers should remove sufficient of the preparation for one treatment on a clean spatula or disposable plastic dish which should be thrown away after use.

Local steroids have revolutionised the treatment of eczema, so some comments will be made on their nature and how they should be used. Hydrocortisone is a naturally occurring hormone and was the first to be used. It is the weakest and is available in lotions, creams or ointments, usually at 1% strength. Steroid preparations of intermediate strength include clobetasone butyrate 0.05% (Eumovate) and flurandrenolone 0.025% (Haelan). There are many strong local steroids; betamethasone BP (Betnovate) and fluocinolone acetonide 0.025% (Synalar) are but two examples. The last mentioned at 0.2% or clobestasol propionate 0.05% (Dermovate) are examples of very strong steroids.

Strong steroids are the best initial treatment for burns, scalds, frostbite or even severe sunburn. They lessen the amount of tissue damage and reduce pain more quickly than anything else, particularly when used in an ointment base. Adding antiseptics such as phenoxyethanol 2% reduces secondary infection. *Pseudomonas aeruginosa* is the main organism with extensive burns, and it is then necessary to use silver nitrate 0.5% with chlorhexidine 0.2% lotion or cream.

Local steroids should be used in the lowest strength that can be guaranteed to completely clear an eczematous eruption. The team should make sure the patient obtains and actually uses sufficient ointment to clear the rash. Steroids are only suppressive so should be continued for up to a fortnight after the skin is clear, thus giving the body time for natural healing and minimising the chance of relapse. Occasional use of the strong ones merely to allay irritation should be discouraged as their effect is cumulative and damage to the skin may occur. This is due to absorption of the drug causing superficial changes in the collagen. The skin becomes waxy and atrophic, feeling thin and smooth to the touch. Telangiectasia develops which takes a year or two to clear, or striae which are disfiguring and permanent. Reticulate areas of purpura may appear after minor trauma to vessels unsupported by normal collagen. The changes are the same as in senile purpura where the collagen has been damaged by the sun's rays over a period of many years. In other words, steroids prematurely age the skin.

Certain sites are more vulnerable than others. Only weak preparations should be used to treat the face, thin skin such as the inner thighs and the young. It is not generally realised that very strong steroids are absorbed in sufficient quantities to cause systemic effects, such as the buffalo hump and moon facies of Cushing's syndrome. Fatalities have occurred. One gram of a very strong steroid ointment may produce the same systemic changes as 1 mg of prednisolone. Repeat prescriptions should not be given without checking the skin for side-effects. The remarkable effectiveness of local steroids must be matched by correct management; be sure of the diagnosis before they are used.

Steroids may suppress the normal inflammatory reaction as for example in a ringworm infection which may then only look like a mild intertrigo. This condition is known as tinea incognito which may be undiagnosed for long periods. Since steroids have been introduced an interesting rosacea-like eruption has been recognised called perioral dermatitis. It is probably due to a very mild seborrhoeic dermatitis being treated with steroids. Weaning from them is quite a problem as cessation causes exacerbation and the patient immediately goes back to them. Oral tetracycline together with topical hydrocortisone and tetracycline is then needed as in the treatment of rosacea. The patient must be warned that the rash will worsen for up to a week, otherwise he will not persist with the treatment.

Avoiding iatrogenic disease

Certain medicaments may be very effective but because of their antigenicity cause sensitivity reactions. This problem has already been discussed in the chapter on dermatitis from page 80. Diseases due to medicines are termed iatrogenic. Rashes caused by ingested drugs are called *dermatitis medicamentosa* while those due to local application *dermatitis venenata*. Streptomycin is a good example of a preparation that can cause either form of dermatitis. It is probably the most effective local application when used as a 2% solution for clearing secondary infection prior to grafting leg ulcers. Unfortunately it readily sensitises the skin and causes the development of antibiotic resistance and should therefore rarely be used. Neomycin is a similar antibiotic which has been chosen by several manufacturers for inclusion in their local steroid preparations. Any sensitisation reaction is then partially masked by the steroid and the duration of the eruption unnecessarily prolonged.

Observations by the nursing staff of any lack of improvement or change for the worse are of fundamental importance in management. It is usually a few days before improvement is noticed but reactions can be produced within hours. Communication with the medical staff should automatically follow any adverse change in the state of the patient's skin or general health.

Anaesthetic ointments are often a source of trouble. They are often applied over long periods for anogenital irritation, frequently in the absence of a correct diagnosis and full examination! They contain benzocaine or its derivatives and are best avoided. Antihistamine creams are cheap and rapidly relieve irritation. Repeated use causes sensitisation, so they should be reserved for self-limiting lesions such as bites or stings. These conditions in any event respond better to the very strong steroids, particularly in alcoholic solution as are available in some scalp applications. Oral antihistamines can be given in addition for quicker relief as they rarely cause iatrogenic disease.

Antibiotics and antiseptics are used more frequently than is necessary. Inflamed skins are often more due to external or internal reactions than to infection. Alternatively, an inflamed rash may become secondarily infected and could then benefit from mild antiseptic treatment. Chemical antiseptics are less likely to cause sensitivity dermatitis or bacterial resistance than antibiotics, but it should not be forgotten that they tend to sting and aggravate an inflamed skin when applied in too strong a concentration. Chemical antiseptics are also the first choice for the treatment of primary infections of the skin. Figure 76 gives a rough guide to some of the more common ones and the organisms against which they are effective.

Removing stains from clothing or one's own skin may sometimes be necessary. The natural tendency is to use solvents at hand, but these may not necessarily be the best for the job or the skin. The ideal cleansing agent should not irritate or sensitise; it should be pleasant to use and

Antiseptics	Organisms				
	Staphylococci	Streptococci	Pseudomonas	Proteus	Candida
Chrystal violet Econazole Clioquinol	+	+	−	+	+
Chlorhexidine Dibromopropamidine	+	+	±	+	±
Silver nitrate Phenoxyethanol	±	±	+	+	−

Fig. 76 Pathogenic organisms and their usual sensitivity to common antiseptics.

easy to apply. Tar can be removed with trichlorethylene, as can the stains of dithranol and usually crystal violet. The last mentioned, as well as silver nitrate stains, can be removed by a solution of sodium thiosulphate 20% (photographic 'hypo'). A weak solution of sulphuric acid may have to be applied beforehand for resistant crystal violet stains and potassium iodide 10% for those from silver. After adopting any of these procedures the skin should be washed with soap and warm water, carefully dried and an emollient cream applied.

Conclusion

The philosophy of therapy is still summarised by Sir Robert Hutchison's prayer of over half a century ago:

From inability to let well alone;
From too much zeal for the new and
  contempt for what is old;
From putting knowledge before wisdom,
  science before art, and
  cleverness before commonsense;
From treating patients as cases and
From making the cure of the disease
  more grievous than
  the endurance of the same,
Good Lord deliver us.

Appendix. Dermatological formulary

Preparations are listed alphabetically except when bracketed into therapeutic groups. The abbreviation BP refers to the *British Pharmacopoeia* and BPC to the *British Pharmaceutical Codex*.

Applications	Therapeutic use
Arachis or cooking oil	Cleaning off pastes
Benzyl benzoate application BP	Scabies
Betamethasone scalp application (Betnovate alcoholic)	⎧ Otitis externa, bites, some scarring alopecias
Clotrimazole 1% alcoholic solution (Canesten)	⎨ Seborrhoea of scalp, otitis externa
Salicylic acid and mercuric chloride lotion BPC	⎩ Seborrhoea of scalp, otitis externa (short-term use only)
Chlorhexidine 0.5% in 70% isopropyl alcohol (also available as swabs)	Preparing skin for injections
Chlorhexidine 0.5% tulle (Bactigras)	Pinch grafting, eroded coccal infections
Crude coal tar BP	Chronic psoriasis
Dihydroxyacetone 5% in industrial methylated spirit	Vitiligo, cosmetic treatment
Glutarldehyde 10% (Glutarol)	Common warts
Idoxyuridine 5% (Herpid)	Herpes zoster and simplex of skin
Phenol, liquefied BP	Pyogenic granulomas and cysts as detailed on page 182
Podophyllin 30% in acetone	Soft warts
Aluminium chloride hexahydrate 20% in absolute alcohol	⎧ Axillary hyperidrosis as detailed on page 125
Propantheline 5–10% (finely powdered from tablets), acetone 50%, in industrial methylated spirit	⎩ Hyperidrosis
Silver nitrate stick	Warts, pyogenic granuloma, excess granulations on leg ulcers, aphthous ulcers
Sodium hypochlorite 0.5% solution (Milton ½ strength) and liquid paraffin in equal quantities	Leg ulcers, bedsores, raw surfaces

Applications (*cont.*)	Therapeutic use
Trichloracetic acid, saturated	Seborrhoeic warts, common warts, xanthelasma with care

Creams

Aqueous cream BP	Bland cream, also as a hand cream
Aqueous calamine cream BP with phenol 2%	Eczematous reactions when becoming drier (less absorption)
Benzoyl peroxide 5% gel	⎰ Acne vulgaris
Dibromopropamidine cream with	⎱ Acne vulgaris, sycosis barbae
precipitated sulphur 10% and	For rosacea the precipitated sulphur
hydrocortisone 2%	should be at 2% strength
Dibromopropamidine cream (Brulidine)	⎰ Surface infections, impetigo, nasal carriage of staphylococci
Chlortetracycline 3% cream	Impetigo, nasal carriage when patient is intolerant to chemical antiseptics
Clobetasone butyrate 0.05% cream (Eumovate) (intermediate strength steroid)	Widespread eczematous reactions
Dithranol 0.25% cream (Dithrocream 0.25%)	Psoriasis of scalp, flexures and thin lesions, pityriasis alba with care
Dithranol 0.5% cream (Dithrocream Forte)	Resistant psoriasis of scalp or flexures
Econazole 1% cream (Ecostatin)	⎰ Seborrhoea, fungi, yeasts, erythrasma
Miconazole 2%, hydrocortisone 1% cream (Daktacort).	Anogenital pruritus, angular stomatitis
Clioquinol 3%, hydrocortisone 1% cream (Vioform hydrocortisone)	Seborrhoea, also anogenital pruritus
Silver nitrate 0.5%, chlorhexidine 0.2% in cetamacragol A cream BP	Leg ulcers, pyocyaneus and proteus infections, bed sores
Titanium dioxide paste 15%, emulsifying ointment 20% in water	Barrier for treatment of actinic dermatoses, treated chronic discoid lupus erythematosus of face
Urea 10% cream (Calmurid)	Tylosis or thick skin (Keratolytic)

Elixirs

Promethazine elixir (Phenergan)	Sedative and antihistaminic for children

Injections

Lignocaine injection 1%	Local infiltration
Lignocaine injection 2%	Nerve block and small biopsies only
Lignocaine 2% and adrenaline injection	Treatment of facial moles only

Injections (*cont.*)
Triamcinolone intradermal 1%

Diazepam 10–20 mg i.m. or i.v.

Lotions
Calamine lotion BP

Calamine lotion with 0.5% crystal
violet
Calamine lotion with phenol 2%
and menthol 1.5%

Calamine lotion with 3% sulphur
Calamine lotion with 10% sulphur
Calamine lotion with 15% sulphur
Malathione 0.5% lotion (Prioderm)
(inflammable preparation)
Padimate A 2.5% alcoholic solution
(Spectraban)
Silver nitrate 0.5%, chlorhexidine
0.2% in water

Ointments (non-steroid)
Benzoic acid compound ointment BP
(Whitfield's ointment)

Calamine and coal tar ointment
BPC with podophyllin 0.1%
Coal tar and salicylic acid ointment
BP

Crotamiton 10% ointment (Eurax)
Crystal violet 0.5%, water 25% in
emulsifying ointment
Dithranol 0.1% in soft paraffin

Dithranol 0.2%, hard paraffin 20%
in soft paraffin
Dithranol 0.5%, salicylic acid 0.5%,
chloroform 2.5%, in equal
quantities of hard, and soft paraffin BP
(Dithrolan) (chrysarobin 5% in
this base gives similar results)

Therapeutic use
Intralesional injection (or pressure
jet) in keloid, granuloma,
granuloma annulare, necrobiosis
lipoidica, chronic discoid lupus
erythematosus, (undertreat to
avoid dimpling)
Uncontrolled tension and irritation

Wet rashes (and neutralising
trichloracetic acid)
Infected wet rashes

Neurotic excoriations, senile
pruritus, papular urticaria, lichen
planus
Rosacea
Acne vulgaris
Acne vulgaris
Lice

Actinic barrier

Intertrigo and leg ulcers due to
pseudomonas (3-hourly soaks)

Fungus infections, but not
anogenital or submammary unless
diluted
Thicker eczema

Psoriasis of scalp, face and guttate
type. Removal of stiff dithranol
ointment from scalp and crude
coal tar from skin
Insect bites, scabies
Artefacts

Dry exfoliative psoriasis (start
cautiously on thickest area)
Thin or flexural psoriasis

Psoriasis, as detailed on page 22
(not for acute spreading or
inflamed psoriasis)

Ointments (non-steroid) (*cont.*)
Stiff dithranol 2% ointment
(prescription otherwise as previous)
Emulsifying ointment BP

Fusidate 2% ointment (Fusidin)

Lignocaine ointment 5%

Nystatin ointment
Oxytetracycline 3%, hydrocortisone
1% ointment (Terra-cortril)

Polymyxin, bacitracin ointment
(Polyfax)
Salicylic acid 20% ointment
Salicylic acid and sulphur (3%)
ointment BP

Yellow soft paraffin BP

Zinc and caster oil ointment BP

Ointments (steroid—weak)
Hydrocortisone 1% ointment BP
Hydrocortisone 1% ointment BP
with phenoxyethanol 2%
(Phenoxytol)
Betamethasone ointment BP 1 part
with 4 parts of calamine and coal
tar ointment BPC (short shelf life)
Betamethasone ointment BP
chlorquinaldol 3% (Steroxin)
ointment titanium dioxide paste
(equal quantities) (short shelf life)

Ointments (steroid—intermediate)
Flurandrenolone 0.0125% ointment
(Haelan)
Triamcinolone in orabase

Therapeutic use
Resistant psoriasis, chronic fungus
of toe clefts
Bland emollient application,
cleansing eczematous skin, for
baths 50 g for sore rashes
Nasal carriage and impetigo, if there
is intolerance to chemicals
After podophyllin treatment for
condylomata only
Moniliasis, chronic paronychia
Wet inflamed rashes, Stevens–
Johnson syndrome, pemphigus
vulgaris, pemphigoid. Steroid
induced rosacea and perioral
dermatitis, with oxytetracycline
Pyocyaneus infections, when there is
intolerance to silver nitrate cream
Strong keratolytic
Seborrhoeic keratoses, seborrhoeic
dermatitis and of scalp, rosacea if
used cautiously and sparingly at
night time with a simple face
cream by day
Acute psoriasis, localising
trichloracetic acid, protection for
nurses' nails
Napkin eruptions

Eczema of face, dry eczema
Pemphigus, pemphigoid

Eczema of face, infantile and
widespread dry eczema

Genital pruritus and eczema

Dry eczema, widespread and
infantile
Mouth ulcers and lichen planus in
the mouth

Ointments (steroid—strong)

Betamethasone ointment BP
(Betnovate) (betamethasone
valerate 0.1%)
Betamethasone ointment BP with
chlortetracycline 3% (Betnovate A)
Betamethasone ointment BP with
crystal violet 0.1%

Betamethasone ointment BP with
crystal violet 0.25% and
phenoxyethanol 2%

Therapeutic use

Eczema (not bacterial or fungal
infections, nor rosacea or
psoriasis)
Pemphigus

Eczema, rapid out-patient treatment,
as a marker and to deter use on
the face
Eczema, rapid in-patient treatment
and with occlusion

Ointments (steroid—very strong)

Clobetasol propionate 0.05%
ointment (Dermovate)

Chronic discoid lupus
erythematosus, lichen sclerosis et
atrophicus, keloid, granuloma
annulare, necrobiosis lipoidica,
sarcoid, pretibial myxoedema
(used accurately)

Paints

Crystal violet 0.5% in water

Staphylococcal infections and under
zinc paste with clioquinol
bandages, in leg ulcers or
gravitational dermatitis, candida,
fungi, erythrasma, chronic
paronychia, biopsy wounds, and
with dithranol for psoriasis as
detailed on page 26

Potassium permanganate 0.5% in
water

Vitiligo, cosmetic treatment.

Pastes

Zinc and salicylic acid paste BP
(Lassar's) with phenoxyethanol
2% (Phenoxytol)
Zinc and coal tar paste BPC (White's
tar paste)

Stasis dermatitis and protection of
surrounding skin when using
silver nitrate soaks
Pruritic and facial psoriasis, removal
of dithranol stains

Pessaries

Econazole
Nystatin

Moniliasis
Moniliasis (pessaries to be sucked
3 times daily in mouth infections)

	Therapeutic use
Plasters Salicylic acid plaster 40% BP	Warts, corns, soft corns
Powders Polynoxylin powder (Anaflex)	Infections, especially in flexures and on penis, with psuedomonas or proteus
Talc dusting powder BP	Used over dithranol ointment
Solutions Potassium permanganate solution 1 in 2500	Baths, pyogenic infections
Saline baths, 1 kg per 100 litres	Sore rashes
Chlorhexidine 0.02% in water	Staphylococcal infections (small baths)
Tablets Azatadine 1 mg (Optimine)	Long-acting potent antihistaminic, containing no colouring
Prednisolone BP 5 mg	⎰ Potentially fatal dermatoses
Azathioprine BP 50 mg	⎱ As above, often used together
Chlorpheniramine BP 4 mg (Piriton)	Quick-action, short-duration potent antihistaminic
Clofibrate BP 500 mg	Xanthomatosis
Dapsone BP 100 mg	Dermatitis herpetiformis
Diazepam BP 5 mg	⎰
Nitrazepam BP 5 mg	⎱ Sedative
Griseofulvin tablets BP 125 mg, 500 mg	Fungi (not monilia, erythrasma, and pityriasis vesicolor)
Hydrocortisone 2.5 mg pellets (Corlan)	Mouth ulcers
Mepacrine hydrochloride BP 100 mg or Chloroquine sulphate BP 200 mg	Discoid lupus erythematosus
Oxytetracycline BP 250 mg	Acne vulgaris, rosacea, steroid induced rosacea and perioral dermatitis
Promethazine BP 10 mg, 25 mg	Long-acting sedative and antihistaminic

Index

Bold type is used to indicate the main references; colour plates (pl.) are listed at the end of each entry. The formulary (pp. 215–20) is not indexed under individual headings.

A

Abscesses 65, 116
Acarus 138–9
Acne vulgaris 63
  other types 65
Actinic reticuloid 88, **89**
Adenoma sebaceum **169**, 181
Adrenaline **71**, 75
Age/exposure changes 77, **156–7**, 170
Alcohol 31, 47, 199
Allergens/antigens 42, 46, 78–86, **91–2**, 212
Alopecia 110, 176, 208
  areata 8, **53**
  diffuse **54**, 89
  male pattern 54
  scarring 56, 101, 121, pl. 34
Anaphylaxis **92**, 135
Angioma 164
  cherry 166
Antibiotics 64, 66, 88, 98, 116, 119
  side-effects 45, 60, 66, 79, 82, 93, 118
Antihistamines 4, 45, **71**
Antiseptics 4, **213**
Artefacts 49
Arthritis, rheumatoid 100, 146
Assessment *see* Caring about patients *and* Nursing observation
Asthma 40, 92
Atopy **40**, 92

B

Balanitis 66

Bandages
  adhesive 46, 49, 88, **148**
  compression **147**, 152, **155**
Barrier cream 59, 86
  actinic **88**, 101
Baths 23
  Sitz 113
  tar 31
Bedbugs 137
Biopsy **178–9**, 187, 189
Bites 135
Blackheads 63–5
Blepharitis, seborrhoeic 61
Blistering diseases 91, **93–9**
Boils 114
Bowen's disease 171
Burns 94, **211**

C

Candida albicans 60, 61, 67, **118**, 190, pl. 25
Carbon dioxide 64, 113, **184**
Carbuncles **114**, 190
Carcinoma
  basal-cell 171, pl. 33
  intraepidermal 171
  squamous-cell 171
Caring about patients 1, 8, 32, 63, 67, 89, 93, 96, 98, 99, 100, 157, 176–7
  terminal 176–7
Cautery 163, 166, **180–1**
Cellulitis 116
Chicken pox 126
Chilblains 146
Chiropody 197
Chondrodermatitis helicis 167

Chronicity 8, 19, 41, 86
  prevention of **4**, 11, 87, 202, 204
Cleansers 4
Clotrimazole 61, 62, 124
Cold sores 126
Condyloma accuminata 132
Consultation **8–9**, 11
Creams 210
  barrier 59, 86
  covering **164**, 168
Fluorouracil 132, **183**
Cross-infection 19, 99, 116, 125,
  149
Cross-sensitivity 72, 74, 78
Cryotherapy 128, 132, 133, 163,
  166, 167, 170, 171, 172, 174,
  183–5
Crystal violet 21, 26, 29, 52, 113,
  120, 149
Curettage 180
Cytotoxic drugs 96, 98, 100, 175,
  176

D

Dandruff 61–2
Dapsone 95
Depression 49, 67
Dermabrasion 185
Dermatitis **76–90**
  contact 2, 75, 76, **78–87**
    differential diagnosis 43,
    70, 81–3, 125
    from chrome 79, 93
    from clothing 79
    from cosmetics 79
    from hair dye 82
    from medicaments 79
    from nickel 43, 79, 84, 93
    from plants 81
    from rubber 79, 83
    in nurses 80
    management 86–7
  exfoliative 72, 88, 89
  herpetiformis **94**, 97
  housewife's 77
  infective eczematoid 114
  medicamentosa 212
  napkin (diaper) 59

Dermatitis (*cont.*)
  perioral 212
  primary irritant 76–8
  seborrhoeic 13, 40, **57–8**, 114
    differential diagnosis 16, 43,
    54
    treatment 87–90
    venenata 212, 213
Dermatomyositis 100, **105**
Diabetes 61, 102, 114, 146, 152,
  160, 197, 199
Diathermy 114, 166, **181**
Diet 58, 64, 159, **197–9**
  elimination 71
Dinitrochlorbenzene 53, 133
Disease *see specific types*
Dithranol **20–6**, 29, 37
  contraindications **20–1**, 38
Dithrolan **29**, 37
Dogger Bank Itch 78
Dressings 1, 20, 23, **32–7**, 87, 112
  occlusive 52
Drug eruptions **72–5**, 103
  types 72–4
  fixed 73

E

Econazole 58, 60, 67, 89, 120, 124,
  176
Eczema **39–47**, 161, 203
  differential diagnosis 16, 39, **43–4**
  exogenous 76, 86, *see also*
    Dermatitis
  gravitational 144, 147
  management 44
  seborrhoeic 57
  secondary absorption 43, 151
  treatment 45–6
  types 40–3, pl. 11, 12
Electromagnetic spectrum 192
Embryology 7, **205**
Emulsifying ointment 20, 31, 44
Erysipelas 116
Erysipeloid 117
Erythema multiforme 73, 92,
  98–9, 126, pl. 19
Erythema nodosum 74, **108**, pl. 21
Erythrasma 67, **117**, pl. 22, 23

F

Favus 121, pl. 34
Fleas 137
Fluoramethane (Freon) 184
Fluorouracil cream 132, **183**
Folliculitis 114
Formulary 215–20
Frostbite 94, **211**
Furunculosis 114

G

Genetics 3, 13, 39, 40, 57, 70, 143
Glandular fever 74
Glossary 248
Gloves, use of **19**, 33, 88, 110, 119, 149
Gluten enteropathy **94**, 199
Granuloma 106
 annulare 125
 pyogenic 167, pl. 31
Gravitational scaling 151, pl. 28
Grenz rays 31, 46, 49, 164, 166, 175, 194, **195–6**
 with psoralens 175, **195**
Griseofulvin 124
Gumma 110

H

Haemangiomas 164
Hair 206, 207
 growth cycle 53, **207**
 permanent waving 207
 transplants 55, **185**
Hayfever 40, 92
Herpes
 simplex 78, **126**
 in eczema 42
 varicella 127
 zoster 127, 176
Histamine 70, 92, 112
Histiocytoma 168
History
 patient's 2, 3, **8**, 11, 17, 19
 suppression **9–10**, 11, 19
Hodgkin's disease 103, **176**

Hydradenitis suppurativa 114
Hydrocortisone injections 135
Hyperidrosis 125
Hypothermia 15, **89**

I

Ichthyosis **40**, 77
IgE and IgG 40, **92**
Immunisation 42, 92, 93, 108
Immunology viii, 79, **91–3**, 105, 106, 111, 112, 114, 116, 118
Impetigo 94, **115–16**
Incubation time 7, 16, 69, 84
Infection
 anaerobic 151
 Gram negative 26, 46, 60, 113, 149
 Gram positive 112, 149
Infestations 135–42
Insight 6, **9–11**, 17, 19, 38, 44, 47, 62, 188
Intertrigo **57–60**, 66, 117, 118, pl. 25

K

Keloid 166
Kerato-acanthoma 169
Keratosis, seborrhoeic 163
 treatment 180, 182
Keratosis, solar **170**, 183, 184, pl. 32
Kerion 121, pl. 26
Koebner's phenomenon 13, 29, 55, 130
Kveim test 109

L

Leishmaniasis 109
Lentigo 168
 malignant 174
Leprosy 106–8
Leukaemia 103, **176**
Leukoplakia 102, **170**
Lice 136–7

Lichen
  planus **55–6**, 200, pl. 13, 14
    differential diagnosis 16, 44,
      55, 72, 101
    sclerosus et atrophicus 102
    simplex 43
Light sensitivity 72, 88
Lipomas 168
Lotions 210
Lupus
  erythematosus
    discoid 100–1, pl. 20
    systemic 100
    vulgaris 108
Lyell's disease 115
Lymphangitis 116
Lymphocytes, B and T   79, **91**
Lymphoedema 117, 144

M

Magenta 120, 124
Malignancy, systemic   96, **102–5**
Melanoma, malignant 172
  differential diagnosis 180, 183
Metastases, skin 176
Methotrexate 31
Metronidazole 67, 151
Miconazole 60, 61, 68, 124
Migraine 40
Milia 181
Miliaria rubra 59
Mites, harvest, food, grain 138
Moles 162–3
Molluscum
  contagiosum 128
  sebaceum 169
Morphea 101
Mouthwash 56
Mycology 189–90
Mycosis fungoides **174–6**, 178,
    193, 196

N

Naevus
  flammeus 164
  spider 166

Nails 45, 206–7
  fungal infection 123
  in exfoliative dermatitis 89
  in lichen planus 56
  in psoriasis 13
  polished 5
Neurodermatitis 43
Neurofibromata 168
Neurotic excoriations **49**, 152
Nitrogen, liquid 184
Nurse
  allocation 2, 18, 21
  community 202
  occupational health 201–2
Nursing management 1–2
Nursing observation   7, 11, 17, 19,
    212

O

Oedema 87, **144**, 147, 152
Oil, cooking 30, 40, 87
Ointments 209–10
  emulsifying 20, 31, 44
Onychogryphosis 157, 197
Organ transplants 91, 93
Otitis externa 61–2

P

Paget's disease of nipple 171
Papular urticaria 135–6
Paraffin, yellow soft 20, 30, 31
Paronychia
  chronic 119–20
  of newborn 115
Pastes 209–10
Patch test 2, 78, 82, 84, **85–6**
  photo 86, 193
Patient allocation 2, **18**, 21
Pavlov's reflex 9
Pediculosis 136–7
Pemphigoid 95–7
Pemphigus 96–8, pl. 18
  neonatorum 116
Petroleum jelly 20, 30, 31
Phenol 114, 128, 132, **182**

Photochemotherapy 192
see also PUVA
Physiotherapy 148–9, **196**
Pill, contraceptive 54, 64
Pinch grafting 152, **186–8**, 190
Pityriasis
  capitis 61–2
  rosea 125–6
  vesicolor **118**, 190
Placebo 200
Poison ivy 81
Polynoxylin 60, 113
Polythene occlusion 46
Pompholyx 42
Port wine stain 164
Potassium permanganate 43, 68,
  88, 113
Pressure jet ('Dermojet') 46, 64,
  166
Prickly heat 59
Primula obconica **81**, 93
Proformas
  gravitational 147, **153–5**
  pinch grafting 186–8
  psoriasis 20, **37–8**
Prurigo 48
Pruritus
  anogenital 10, 44, **66–7**, 118, 137
  generalised 102–3, 105, 176
  senile **103**, 157
Pseudomonas aeruginosa 62, 99,
  144, 211
Psoriasis 3, 9, **12–38**, 67, 193,
  pl. 1–10
  causes **12–13**, 16
  differential diagnosis **15–16**, 44,
    54, 55, 117–18
  management 17
  prognosis 10, 17, 22
  treatment **19–38**
    exfoliative and pustular 31–2
  types 13–15
Purpura 103, 105, 176
  anaphylactoid (Henoch
    Schonlein) 93
  senile **156**, 211
PUVA, also psoralens 32, 81,
  174–5, **192–4**
  complications 194
  with dithranol 194

R

Raynaud's phenomenon 101
Relationships
  interpersonal 3, **9**, 11, 16, 18, 39
  patient/nurse/doctor vii, 18
Rhinitis, allergic 40
Rhinophyma 66, 185
Ringworm 67, **120–5**
  differential diagnosis 16, 43, 54,
    123, 125
  treatment 124–5
Rodent ulcer 171, pl. 33
Rosacea 7, **65–6**, 185, pl. 15, 16

S

Salabrasion 185
Sarcoidosis 108–9
Scabies 138–42
Scleroderma
  localised 101
  systemic 101
Seborrhoea 57–68
  see also Dermatitis, seborrhoeic
Serum sickness 93
Shingles 127, 176
Silver nitrate 26, 60, 113, 149, 209
Sites of emotional expression 67
Skin, structure and function 205–7
Smallpox 128
Sores, pressure 148, **158–9**, pl. 30
Stains
  removing of 23, 30, **213–14**
  protection 19, 149
Staphylococci 45, 65, **112–13**, 115,
  119, 121, 149, 191
Steroids
  intralesional 46, 49, 64
  systemic 71, 89, 96, 98, 100
Steroids, local 211–12
  and dermatitis 87, 89, 90
  and eczema 45–6
  and lupus erythematosus 101
  and prurigo 49
  and seborrhoeic affections 60–2
  side-effects 21, 31, 74, 94, 112,
    211–12, pl. 16
  weaning from 31

Stevens-Johnson syndrome   73,
    98–9, pl. 19
Stockings, elastic   148
Stomatitis, angular   61
Streptococci   116–17
Stress
  causes   3, 8, 9, 11, **63**
  effects of 4, 7, 8, 16, 40, 44, 49,
    51, 53, 54, 55, 57, 62, 65, 67,
    70, 71, 103, 126, 198
  secondary   **19**, 55, 63, 66, 89,
    144, pl. 34
Sycosis barbae   61
Syphilis   109–11
Systemic rashes   100–5

T

Tags, skin   163, 185
Tar   20, **26–9**
  preparations   25, 26, 30, 31, 46,
    49, 87
Target organ   **3**, 39, 49
Tattoos   185
Team   1, 5, 10, 11, 160, **200–4**
Therapy   2–4
Thrombophlebitis   147, 158
Thrush (candidiasis)   118–19, pl. 25
Tinea
  capitis   121, pl. 24, 26
  corporis   121
  cruris   121, pl. 27
  incognito   212
  pedis   121–3
Tongue, geographical   40
Toxic epidermal necrolysis   115
Tranquillisers   **4**, 19, 45, 49, 52, 56,
    160
Transport medium   191
Treatment
  principles of   209–11
  teaching   2, 18, 20, 22, 45
Trichloracetic acid   163, **181–2**
Trichomonas   67
Trichotillomania   53
Tuberculosis   108
Tuberose sclerosis   169

U

Ulcers
  arteriosclerotic   145–6
  gravitational   **143–4**, 199, pl. 29
    management   147–55
    tracing   151–2
    varicose   143–4
Ultraviolet light   31, 63, 76–7, 113,
    192–4
Urticaria   40, **69–70**, 92
  management   70–1

V

Varicose ulcers   143–4
    see also   Ulcers, gravitational
Verrucae   130–4
Vicious circle   **4**, 11, 39, 44, 66
Virology   191
Von Recklinghausen's disease   168

W

Warts   130–4
  seborrhoeic   163
Whitfield's ointment   124
Wickham's striae   55
Wigs   55
Wood's lamp   117, **120**, pl. 23, 24
Worker, medical-social   201

X

Xanthomata   **102**, 182, 199
X-ray treatment   46, 120, 166, 169,
    194–5

Y

Yoghurt   64, 118